I0198603

Cracking Chests

How Thoracic Surgery
Got from Rocks to Sticks

—⁂—

Alex G. Little, M.D.

Cracking Chests, published November, 2022

Editorial and proofreading services: Beth Rapps; Gina Sartirana

Interior layout and cover design: Howard Johnson

Photo Credits: Cover: Lungs, csp27962983 by sciencepics; www.canstockphoto.com

Figure 8: Reprinted with permission from the Journal of the American College of Surgeons, formerly Surgery Gynecology & Obstetrics.

Author Photo courtesy of Louise Little

All other images owned by Alex G. Little, M.D.

SDP Publishing

Published by SDP Publishing, an imprint of SDP Publishing Solutions, LLC.

The characters, events, institutions, and organizations in this book are strictly fictional. Any apparent resemblance to any person, alive or dead, or to actual events is entirely coincidental.

All rights reserved. No part of the material protected by this copyright notice may be reproduced or utilized in any form or by any means, electronic or mechanical, including photocopying, recording, or by any information storage and retrieval system, without written permission from the copyright owner.

To obtain permission(s) to use material from this work, please submit an email request with subject line: SDP Publishing Permissions Department. Email: info@SDPPublishing.com.

ISBN-13 (print): 979-8-9862833-0-2

ISBN-13 (ebook): 979-8-9862833-1-9

Library of Congress Control Number: 2022914543

Copyright © 2022, Alex G. Little

Printed in the United States of America

To Louise

Table of Contents

Preface

My chief aim in *Cracking Chests* is to tell the tale of the origins and developments of chest surgery; to follow the passage of one surgical specialty, thoracic surgery, from infancy to maturation. This is less a formal history than the story of the events and surgeons that made a difference. Most books that explore the evolution of surgical thought and practice were written for a medical or even a solely surgical audience. This book differs. It may engage surgeons and other physician readers; however, my priority is a book which is accessible to all readers.

As a chest surgeon, I want the reader to appreciate not just the "facts" but the personal element: what and who was responsible for the incremental development of chest surgery. Earlier books have been written about specific surgeons (*The Knife Man* about John Hunter, and *Genius on the Edge* about William Halsted come to mind), about patient experiences, and other surgical specialties, but none focus on chest surgery as this book does. I think it's time.

Thoracic surgery was built on primitive and tentative surgical advances and only blossomed when necessary prerequisites such as anesthesia and antisepsis matured. I have used my own experiences—the four years of medical school, residency training, and career in academic thoracic surgery—to illustrate what it means to be part of this profession and culture. How are today's thoracic surgeons trained, what diseases do they treat, what's it like to be part of this profession? Accordingly, there are reminiscences from my training, practice, and patient encounters woven into stories of the origins and development of thoracic surgery. One of my goals is to infuse the past with an immediacy and relevance that can be lost in more single-minded histories—to link historical events with modern clinical practices.

The *thorax*, the chest, is the realm of thoracic surgeons who practice thoracic surgery. What are surgeons doing when they operate inside a chest? How were these operations developed? What were the challenges and how were they surmounted? What do the "rocks and sticks" in the title have to do with these things? This book answers questions like these for the curious lay reader, especially those who have personally experienced, or had a friend or relative need, a chest operation. Viewers of TV shows featuring surgeons will be intrigued to learn that the real life of surgery, past and present, is equally full of drama and intrigue.

There is something literally visceral about the reaction to and curiosity about the operations that constitute surgery and the people who perform them. It is a challenge to picture being a participant in an operation; to envisage what it's like to take a scalpel and cut open a chest to remove a cancerous lung. Are you even certain what the esophagus is, what purpose it serves, and how it functions in the act of swallowing? I doubt that imagination is lacking but the necessary background is harder to come by. This is why I want the reader to get a sense of what thoracic surgeons do and how chest surgery got to its present state.

Part of my motive is to bring recognition to the remarkable pioneering people who persisted in the face of societal, religious, and technical challenges. They impacted their specialty, and health care in general, in ways revealed through the fascinating—occasionally astonishing—details of their lives and accomplishments. We would not have our current panoply of surgical capabilities without their efforts. Without the evolution from primitive and hesitant beginnings (using sharpened rocks), to the mature manifestation of chest surgery we enjoy today with minimally invasive surgeons (wielding long, stick-like instruments), cancers of the lung and esophagus would be, as they historically were, routinely and quickly fatal.

"Cracking chests" is medical slang for chest operations, and this book recounts both my own experiences, those of earlier chest surgeons, and fleshes out the origins and evolution of the specialty. Who were the field's pioneer surgeons? I look at their lives, in and out of the operating room, and their struggles to imagine, and then develop, surgical insights they transformed into operative techniques they could ultimately use to treat diseases of the chest such as lung and esophageal cancer. Advances were typically incremental. Failures and errors of judgment and technique litter the surgical road.

Too, the men (women in surgery are a recent—and welcome—addition to the profession, and therefore underrepresented in this story) who developed chest operations were embedded in their time and culture and handicapped by the typically rudimentary condition of medical science. For example, religious dogma for millennia retarded the ability to dissect humans to develop an accurate anatomic map. Absent that basic knowledge, surgical advances were severely slowed. In addition, major, i.e., invasive, surgical procedures were unimaginable before general anesthesia: no awake patient could tolerate the pain and trauma of lengthy procedures inside the body. Early surgeons faced the challenge of writhing patients, creating moving targets and the need to complete operations before the patient died of shock.

This is a selective history, not meant to be comprehensive. My choices of material to include were made based on the diseases I have been particularly interested in and the operations I performed. I have chosen to highlight those surgeons and surgical accomplishments that strike me as being intrinsically interesting and have made a significant and lasting impact on the profession and culture of thoracic surgery. Surgeons on the faculty of medical schools teach and mentor students and residents. They are also responsible for developing advances in the surgical sciences and sharing them with others in the field through presentations at professional meetings and publications in surgical journals. I was fortunate to spend my surgical career in this culture of academia, characterized by curiosity and professionalism. Several of the highlighted surgeons were mentors in my training and became colleagues. In turn, they knew the generation of surgical leaders who preceded them, providing me with secondhand contact with these early practitioners of chest surgery. These experiences have been invaluable as a way to appreciate the thoughts, motives, and inspirations of the men who were the early, even pioneer, surgeons. Today's chest surgeons are standing on the shoulders of these giants.

Finally, I acknowledge two possible criticisms. One is that the included surgeons are all white males. This is a result of the times under discussion and exposes an early medical and societal bias. One of the most positive recent changes both in the medical profession at large and its surgical component is a move to true diversity, including the greatly increased presence of women and people of color. When a similar book is written in the future, females and physicians of color will be seen to have played important roles as they take their rightful place in all of medicine.

This book focuses almost entirely on events in the Western world. The Eastern and Western surgical communities only began to interact and communicate effectively over the past few decades; the beginnings and evolution of surgery in the West were mainly in ignorance of, and uninfluenced by, events elsewhere.

Chest surgery was a blunt instrument for most of recorded history. Now surgeons routinely perform operations for cure of dread cancers and improvement of patients' quality of life. This evolution was not by happenstance. I lived through much of this transition and am sure you will find the drama of this process as engrossing as I have.

I have not "dumbed down" the material but I realize that medical and surgical terminology may collide with reading ease and at times lay terminology is more reasonable. However, some use of anatomical, medical, and physiological language is unavoidable and desirable. Accordingly, there are three appendices for the reader: Appendix One is a Glossary providing frequently used anatomic and medical/surgical terminology used by the medical profession to enable precise communication. I italicized these terms the first time they appeared in the text. I think some sense of the anatomic location of the discussed structures and their relationship to the others should add a useful perspective for the reader. Overviews of chest and esophageal anatomy are provided in Appendices Two and Three. Appendix Three also contains some explanation and depiction of how the esophagus functions and how we test patients to determine the benefit of operative intervention.

Acknowledgments

I am grateful to many teachers and colleagues who did their best to inform me with knowledge, judgment, and technical skills both with words and example during my times as a medical student, surgical resident, and faculty member. These experiences are indelible and informed my book throughout. I acknowledge and am thankful for the Johns Hopkins and University of Chicago surgery faculty who were role models I emulated. I especially thank David Skinner, my Chairman at the University of Chicago, who stimulated me to focus on general thoracic surgery and supported my career both in Chicago and afterward. Ronald Belsey, a pioneer thoracic surgeon, was a consummate thoracic surgeon whose tales of his previous experiences with surgical greats stimulated my interest in the development of our specialty. Tom DeMeester patiently helped me learn and develop surgical skills and an academic platform for thoracic surgery. Of course, all the faculty and residents with whom I worked left their influence, for which I am grateful.

While I taught and mentored medical students and surgical residents, I also learned from them and benefited from the shared experiences. Working together through difficult surgical challenges strengthened us all.

The staff of the library of the University of Arizona School of Medicine received my frequent trips and requests with aplomb and always were helpful, friendly, and encouraging. I am appreciative of their assistance.

My book benefited greatly from the editing skills of Beth Raps. She rescued writing mishaps and her advice and persistent encouragement kept me going. Lisa Akoury-Ross served essential roles as agent and publisher, all with professionalism and good cheer. I thank them both.

More personally, I express my profound gratitude to my dear wife Louise. There would be no book without her. She was my invaluable IT support and Word guru. Most importantly, her encouragement and continual support kept me at work and saw me through the process. She is my motivation and polestar.

Introduction

At the beginning they weren't thoracic surgeons; they weren't surgeons; they weren't even physicians. The earliest "cutters" were simply people trying to help their fellow humans. Accordingly, I use the terms "thoracic surgery" and "thoracic surgeons" to describe them as broad, technically inaccurate, ways to speak of those attempting to deal surgically with diseases of the chest. Eventually these designations acquired their current meaning. The story of thoracic surgery is replete with surgeons who exhibited insight and had enough courage, stamina, and boldness to persist in following their instincts and irrepressible desire to attack diseased organs despite disappointing initial results. You might even call these actions rash: imagine cutting into a patient in the times of immature anesthetic capabilities and the absence of blood transfusions, antiseptic technique, and antibiotics. While their behavior may seem to us now to border on reckless, it was the action of inventive, resourceful, and well-intentioned surgeons who sought to cure cancer or modify malfunctioning organs, and thereby extend or improve the quality of patients' lives.

There was plenty of drama, even though, without television, newspapers, and the Internet, most of the world had no knowledge of these early thoracic surgical efforts. The first generations of pioneers had to ask and answer formidable questions. What happens if you cut and divide this blood vessel? Can a person live with only one lung? If you remove part of the esophagus, what do you replace it with? How these questions, the answers to which made today's operations possible, were answered will interest and surprise.

As for me, I am a thoracic surgeon who spent my career as a faculty member of a medical school. While there were some limited and superficial chest surgery-type activities in remote times, most of the true surgical activities, in the sense of actual operations on internal structures, have taken place in surprisingly recent years. My training and practice overlapped with some of these developments. However, to appreciate early surgical development, it's necessary to understand how anesthesia, techniques for patient ventilation, and antisepsis came about.

Thoracic surgery is chest surgery, the art of performing operations inside the thorax, or chest cavity. Cardiac surgery thrived in the 1970s, when coronary artery bypass surgery became commonplace and its frequency exploded. Thoracic surgery became identified as cardiothoracic surgery. Thoracic surgery is the correct identification. It houses two subspecialties. Cardiac surgery is the discipline practiced by surgeons who operate on the heart and its great blood vessels—the aorta carrying blood to the body and the *pulmonary* artery to the lungs. These surgeons meticulously suture heart or blood vessel tissues, for example, while performing a coronary artery bypass, or repairing or replacing a heart valve.

The other discipline within thoracic surgery is general thoracic surgery. This is the home for surgeons who operate inside the chest but not on the heart. We deal with diseases of a number of chest organs: lungs, esophagus, the *mediastinum* (the middle of the chest between the lungs), the network of intrathoracic nerves, and the *pleura*, a membrane which lines the inside of the chest wall and envelops the lungs. This is my surgical focus. Most of my and my colleagues' surgical activities involve dissecting a cancerous organ free from surrounding tissue and removing it or rearranging anatomic structures. An example of this activity is taking out part of a lung due to lung cancer.

All thoracic surgeons today train in both subspecialties; many practice both. Yet the trend today is for thoracic surgeons, especially academic surgeons who are teaching faculty in medical schools, to focus on one subspecialty. This reduces the potential variety of the surgeon's activities, but it's an inevitable response to the ever-accelerating pace of surgical development akin to advances in the electronic world as described by Moore's law. Technology available for use in operations, and our understanding of the biology of disease, are evolving at an increasingly rapid pace. Surgeons must keep current with these developments to perform at a state-of-the-art level. Practicing *one* of the two subspecialties allows the surgeon to come closer to complete mastery of a field rather than attempt two diverse surgical activities.

I've spent the majority of my career as a general thoracic surgeon regularly performing operative procedures once considered too dangerous or even technically unachievable. The developments in my field are owed to the pioneering surgeons who are the subjects of this book. Their accomplishments and failures are considered in the context of their times and cultures. I have linked them to my own experiences and encounters on my personal journey as a thoracic surgeon to connect chapters and provide a look at what life in this specialty is like.

Surgery is an invasive specialty. Thoracic surgical operations require the surgeon's hands, instruments, or both, to take hold of organs inside the rib cage. The goal, typically, is to remove all or part of one of these organs—or to alter their structure and function in a way beneficial to a patient's quality of life. Gaining access to these organs by an incision in the chest wall [typically between the ribs but occasionally through the sternum (breastbone)] was required during most of history. For nearly all of my practice years, before today's ability to perform operations through small incisions with video camera guidance, we general thoracic surgeons gained access into the chest using an operative approach called a "thoracotomy." This thoracotomy or chest incision, described below, is from *thorax*, the chest, and *-otomy*, to open.

As Figure 1A depicts, in preparation for a thoracotomy, the patient is typically balanced on the operating table lying on one side, with the surgeon facing the chest. In this example, the patient is on

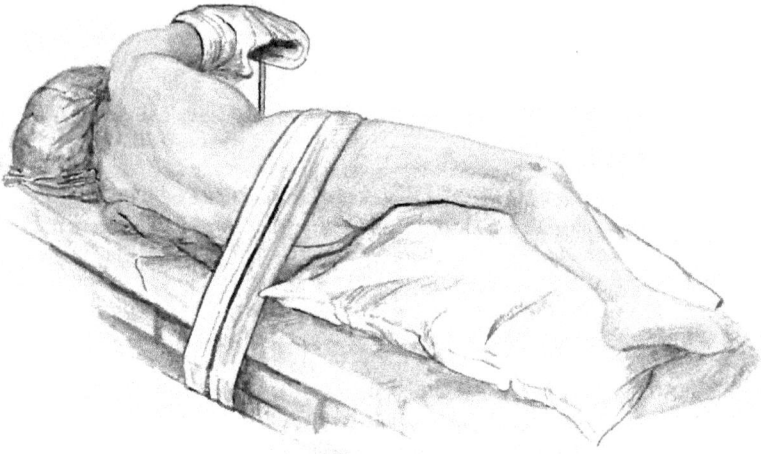

FIGURE 1A.

his left side with his right arm out, supported on a sling. The patient's right chest is fully exposed and the surgical incision in the skin of the right chest is parallel to the ribs, midway between the armpit and hip. This location surprised many of my patients who expected a vertically oriented cut across several ribs. A cut like that would be a poor choice, as severing several ribs would destabilize the chest wall and cause more pain by traumatizing more of the intercostal ("inter-rib") nerves.

   The incision you see in Figure 1B is for what is termed a "lateral thoracotomy," the most frequently chosen location for a chest opera-tion. Beneath the skin, the surgeon cuts through underlying tissues, chest wall muscles, and, ultimately, the muscles bridging the two adjacent ribs. A metal retractor is placed in this gap, and the ribs are stretched apart to expose the chest contents. The subsequent opera-tion through this access is called an "open operation" as the surgeon spreads the ribs apart and the chest is widely opened.

   Thankfully for patients, this type of incision and the open thora-cotomy, though the standard approach for many years, are being supplanted by what is called a "minimally invasive thoracoscopic operation." Although the open thoracotomy served the surgeon well, it was quite painful for the patient. Now the more typical way to get inside a patient's chest is for the surgeon to create a few (typically three or four) small skin incisions used to insert instruments and a video camera to allow the surgeon to perform the operation with less cutting of tissue, particularly muscle, and no stretching ribs apart. The patient has less pain and recovers more rapidly. This is an important advance in surgery. I'll talk about this in more detail further on in the book.

A well-conducted chest operation is an artistic undertaking (not to argue that every surgeon is a Monet). The title of my book comes from non-surgeon physicians' friendly (or snarky) rivalry with us surgeons, under which "cracking chests" in the old, open manner is a clearly barbaric activity, and a brutal beginning to patients' experiences. My perspective is that incising and taking on the responsibility of entering a patient's chest is an elegant and precise undertaking, performed to extirpate and cure a cancer or correct a benign (in the sense of non-cancerous) pathologic condition.

Descriptions of my patients are composite examples drawn from my personal experiences. None of the individuals discussed in the book are based on a specific patient, and I have changed all identifying details in the composite examples to protect the privacy of actual patients.

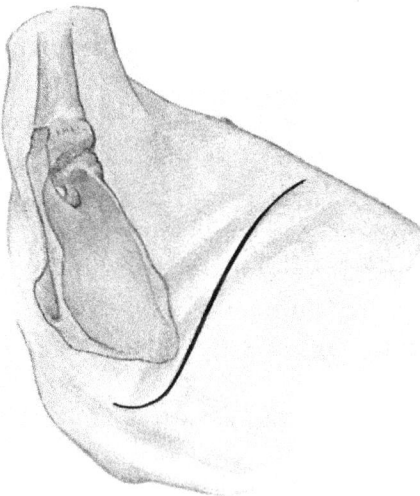

FIGURE 1B.

1

MEDICAL SCHOOL

I followed a circuitous route into medicine and thoracic surgery. I was fortunate to spend my early years in Valdosta, a small southern Georgia town. Valdosta was afloat in a sea of pine trees, which fueled the production of naval stores. These are not where one might purchase a battleship. Naval stores are the components of pine trees used in the construction of wooden sailing ships.

In 1988, a *Sports Illustrated* article about our successful high school football team accurately described ours as a town with "both charm and a certain vitality ... the sort of town that, when you drive through, you think: Now this would be a good place to raise a family." It lacked today's array of entertainment options—television had three channels, if you could get them with your rotary antenna on the roof—but it was safe; families rarely locked their doors. As kids we played (and sweated in the hot, humid air) outside, unsupervised and unworried in the rural countryside. The importance of the football team, and insight into our coach's character, are illustrated by what happened when civil rights came to Valdosta in 1964. Integration in our Deep South town proceeded reasonably smoothly because the Coach was immediately willing to start and play the best athlete, regardless of color.

My father and his father were both general surgeons. Following in their footsteps seems inevitable now but it was far from a sure thing at the time. I stubbornly resisted my ancestral influences. After high school, I eased through the University of North Carolina with no goal in sight. I enjoyed my time but never really applied myself academically. My GPA was as mediocre as you would expect. I graduated in 1965 when the Vietnam War and its attendant draft were in full swing. Like many of my peers, I was not eager to participate in a war with uncertain and debatable goals. However, rather than submit to the vagaries of the draft (or flee the country), I opted for Naval Officers Candidate School which launched me to serve on a shore staff in Hawaii responsible for preparedness for submarine warfare.

Being thousands of miles from home and free to make decisions in a neutral setting, medicine began to attract. I'm not certain what woke me up. Like the later choice of thoracic surgery for my specialty, this was not a rational and carefully thought-out commitment, but seemingly arose from the depths of my subconscious, apparently where I had been keeping a lid on it. All was far from settled, however. I lacked the science courses necessary for admission to medical school, and my graduating grade point average was nowhere near a competitive level. These deficiencies were redressed by a monastic year and a half of pre-med study at UNC after leaving the Navy. My academic performance was sufficient for the eventual admission to the Johns Hopkins School of Medicine in 1970.

I arrived in Baltimore a little full of myself—medical school, Hopkins no less. I was also simply nervous—medical school, Hopkins no less. The adage that you should be careful what you wish for suddenly had meaning. Although the tradition of medical schools routinely failing substantial numbers of entering students was ending, it was still engrained in medical student mythology. It didn't help when I learned that the majority of my classmates—competition as I first thought— were from Ivy League institutions. One has since won the Nobel Prize; at least one other is legitimately competitive for that honor.

It turned out, happily, that times really had changed. Classes began, I settled in, and my adrenalin levels subsided to normal as I realized that medical schools had evolved their philosophy regarding entering students. As remains the case now, once students got through the rigorous admissions process, the goal was to shepherd all to the finish line. Not finishing is now seen as failure of both student and school. In addition, my classmates, while as impressively smart as advertised, were a varied and interesting group, and the atmosphere was collegial and supportive. Although we all wanted to do well, there was very little competition. What do you call the student who graduates last in their medical school class? "Doctor." We were not yet aware that, while class rank and academic standing played no role in acquiring the "M.D.," it would affect competitiveness for residency programs.

I didn't think much of it at the time but there was a spectrum of personalities in my class, and both racial and gender diversity in the student body. This would not be newsworthy today but in 1970, Hopkins was quite different from the norm in this regard. While Hopkins had always admitted some women (as required by an agreement with a women's philanthropic group that raised money to help establish the school in the late 1800s), I had the sense this mandate had been honored somewhat grudgingly over the years. The famous writer Gertrude Stein, for example, was admitted to Hopkins's medical school, but was soon advised it wasn't for her; she departed for a literary life. The movement toward equality had begun by the time I got to Hopkins. My class included women and African Americans. The trend toward representative diversity has continued nationally; now, half or more of the students in medical schools across the country are women, and people of color are more equitably represented.

The four years of medical school were so absorbing that I found them remarkably enjoyable, more pleasure than work. The first two years resembled previous school experiences: lectures in classrooms. I soon fell into a rhythm. Classes took up most of the day Monday through Friday. Nights were for study of textbooks and notes hastily scribbled during the lectures. (A distraction we all appreciated was when one of us slipped a racy slide into a professor's slide deck. Not possible now that PowerPoint is here.) Weekends were for review of the week's material; there was also time for Friday night basketball games and social activities as friendships developed. One of the perks

I most appreciated was the ability to purchase tickets to Baltimore professional sports teams at cut-rate student prices. These were the best of the best: The Colts, Bullets, and Orioles all won championships during my four years.

This was the basic science phase of the curriculum, and I found the material fascinating. Courses focused on anatomy, histology, *physiology,* and pathology (in other words: where organs are, their composition at the cellular level, how they function, and what can go wrong). My mindset began to shift from my undergraduate years. I realized this knowledge was going to be my framework for providing care for my future patients—it was no longer just about regurgitating memorized facts for the purpose of passing tests. Many diseases are named for the physician who identified them; many parts of the body are named for the anatomist who described them. As their eponyms multiplied, I began to feel a connection to these early medical giants. In addition, the faculty were an impressive group. They were mainly laboratory scientists who spent most of their time carrying out basic biomedical research and seemed to have an encyclopedic knowledge of their respective fields. Several of my instructors have made seminal contributions to the understanding of biological or pathological processes and were awarded the Nobel Prize in Medicine or Physiology. I was in awe of their seemingly unlimited store of facts and appreciated their energy and strong, genuine passion for their research. They exuded enthusiasm. Most also displayed a sense of perspective and a self-deprecating humor which, given their obvious stature, diminished our own temptation to take ourselves too seriously.

I was eager for the final two years of medical school, the clinical years. It was a significant change from my past routine, developed over many school years, to get up in the morning, put on a white coat with pockets bulging with a stethoscope and books, and head for the hospital or outpatient clinic rather than a classroom. It was daunting at first. I was certain that patients would quickly identify me as a novice. I became more comfortable as time went by. Less nervous as my experiences grew, I found that patients, despite sickness or anxiety, tolerated me as I took their history and examined them. Students had few real responsibilities; we were there to learn. While the residents and attending physicians were working, I was able to sit and talk to patients, and develop relationships and empathy as I learned what it was like to be around the seriously ill.

In our third year, we broke into small groups for rotations through the clinical specialties of medicine, surgery, pediatrics, obstetrics/gynecology, and psychiatry. (The disciplines of family practice and emergency medicine did not yet exist as specialties.) I was starting to feel like a doctor, finally helping to care for but mainly learning from actual patients—under the tutelage of both residents and the faculty physicians, frequently referred to as the attending physicians. Students were assigned to teams of the supervising residents who were responsible for patients, under the leadership of attending physicians. My earlier premonition came true; I recognized the value of the classroom information acquired during the preceding two years as I became involved with real patients and situations. Patients lingered much longer in the hospital than is the case now, so I spent evenings reading about the patients' diseases and could visit repeatedly to hear firsthand from those afflicted to flesh out the textbook descriptions.

In addition to providing opportunities to learn, these clinical experiences delivered something else of major importance: exposure to the specialty disciplines, the physicians and their patients. Like me, most of my classmates had not yet chosen their final professional specialty; these third-year rotations were our opportunity to find our ultimate niche by sampling career alternatives. We trailed along on hospital rounds in the conga line headed by the faculty physician who led the way from room to room, followed by the senior and junior residents, with us at the tail end. It didn't always go according to plan. A favorite memory is following an attending physician into the wrong patient's room; we couldn't exit until the entire serpentine contingent followed, coiled around, reversed course, and sequentially followed him out without a word to the clueless patient. Perhaps he imagined we had arranged a parade for his benefit.

I wasn't just absorbing information. Learning from passionate and exceptional faculty and residents and sharing their obvious enjoyment of their particular disciplines was seductive and made all choices of specialty attractive—with the caveat that whichever a student chose, it was likely to be for life. It is nearly impossible, after years of practicing one specialty, to simply move to another. This is even more the case now with the advent of numerous subspecialties. I knew I had to decide by the end of the third year or, at the latest, very early in the fourth, as applications for residency programs were submitted in the fall of the fourth year.

The time spent with this variety of physicians and practice specialties made it evident that medicine and its practitioners are not a monolithic mass. During each rotation, students usually developed enough of a friendship with our teachers, especially the residents with whom we spent most of our time, that candid conversation naturally followed. It became clear that not only were they happy practicing their chosen specialty, but they were also confident *their* discipline was elite, as were its practitioners.

Confidence in oneself is a good thing. Actually, it's essential for a doctor who must make life or death decisions. Unfortunately, as the years went by, I observed that while this pervasive mindset was usually harmless, occasionally it led to a rivalry between practitioners which played out generally in a friendly fashion but could lapse into nearly hostile interactions. (As mentioned in the Introduction, this interspecialty interaction led to the usually friendly, occasionally snarky, expression, "cracking chests.") Perhaps this is only an inevitable aspect of the hard-wired competitive side of human nature: it's the "our team is the best" instinct.

As I spent time with the Hopkins faculty, I got insight into the lifestyle they were so enthused about. I saw them shuttle back and forth between their basic science or clinical research activities and their patients. I began to appreciate this ability to meld clinical practice with a research enterprise of one's own and sensed that my practice specialty might not be the only question I needed to answer; choosing between the private practice of surgery and an academic career might also be necessary. Yet I did not give serious consideration to this choice until well into my surgical residency.

I found the challenge of choosing a clinical specialty to be particularly difficult. All had some appeal but my insight into each specialty was limited by my observer status. While students were ostensibly part of the physician team, we were not part of the decision-making process. We were occasionally asked to provide our assessment of a patient. More frequently we were grilled about our knowledge (the so-called Socratic method). I don't know what the experience was like with Socrates, but it stimulated me to be prepared by reading textbooks and medical articles. (Today's students regularly search the Internet as a quick supply of answers in real time to these questions; printed sources can be used later for more in-depth understanding.) Only occasionally did the questioner swerve into condescension to demean us when our answer was not forthcoming.

We were not really responsible for patients. A medical student, even one considering surgery, wasn't asked to take a knife in hand and complete an operation. Without a "hands-on" experience, and even though I earlier had resisted the influence of my father and grandfather, I surprised myself by emerging from the third year with a feeling surgery was *it*. To get additional exposure, I spent a month early in my fourth year of med school immersed in the surgical culture as an "acting intern." I was able to have this experience because Hopkins allowed the students much elective time in the fourth year. Many of us seized the opportunity to be further exposed to possible career choices. For me, this immersion in the "real thing," though short, was enough to bolster my confidence.

As far as the residents were concerned, during my month as an acting intern, I was one of them, a true intern, although I was paired with a resident who kept a close eye and provided guidance. Despite early morning and late evening patient rounds sandwiched around busy days in the operating room, I found I was energized and excited, not fatigued. In the operating room, I enjoyed the rituals and ambiance: donning scrubs, doing the gloving dance with the nurses. More importantly I observed and participated in the conduct of operations carried out by calm and precise surgeons. My role was limited, nothing major; I performed the traditional student role of holding retractors to expose the operative field for the surgeon. But I felt personally involved. Being closer to patients than ever helped me develop empathy for them and learn what postoperative complications, such as infections of the wound, to be alert for. I felt all signs were encouraging; I was in the right place.

In my role as an acting intern, during operations I was mesmerized by the hands of the operating surgeons as they carefully identified tissue planes, dissected into them to separate adjacent tissues and extracted a diseased or cancerous organ. It was captivating, nearly sensual. Physicists and mathematicians speak of the beauty of mathematical equations while most of us just see numbers. They resonate to a chord unheard by us (or at least by me). This was exactly my esthetic reaction to an expertly performed operation.

There was more. My acting internship emphasized to me that a surgeon's activities and responsibilities were not confined to the operating room. When outside of the operating room, surgeons cared for their patients' medical problems such as blood pressure control, diabetes, and respiratory failure. A surgeon could be a complete physician; she or he was not limited to being a technician in the operating room. Projecting these activities over a lifetime was considerably more attractive to me than the prospect of seeing a series of patients in an office.

My final observation was more subjective: surgeons were the physicians with whom I shared the most personality traits and characteristics. One, admittedly, is limited patience. When you operate, the effect on the patient is usually immediate, although admittedly not always positive. There is no waiting to see if, for example, a medication will actually work. I also liked hanging out with surgeons. In today's parlance, they were my people; there was a genuine camaraderie. I figured it was likely I would enjoy doing what they do.

Malcolm Gladwell in *Outliers* suggests that work satisfaction for some is dependent on the complexity of the professional activities, and the questions they ask of a person. I feel the lure of the challenge to master the skills required of a surgeon played a major role in my career choice even if I was not conscious of this at the time. I think this, more than any supposed financial reward, explains why the specialties are attractive to so many graduating medical students. As for many of my critical life decisions, my attraction to surgery was irresistible and visceral. As *The Little Prince* puts it, "In the face of an overpowering mystery, you don't dare disobey."

Surgery and I had chosen each other—now two steps remained. I needed to secure a surgery residency position and complete the remainder of the final school year. I applied to several residency programs and interviewed during the fall. I couldn't find anything to beat the Hopkins program. There were and are other excellent residencies, but it was irresistible to stay home, and happily that worked out. For the remaining school year, it made sense to me to select experiences that would help me take care of patients; I had the remainder of my life to learn to operate. There were no required rotations in the fourth year, so I chose to spend the remaining time learning more about the treatment of patients with infections, heart disorders, high blood pressure, kidney failure, and endocrine disorders. I was preparing myself to care for patients, not just operate on them.

2

EARLY SURGERY

Four years earlier, I was pleased simply to have gotten into medical school. Now I was on the brink of becoming a surgeon. This profession and its culture had been in existence, in the big picture, for only a short time. This chapter explores the questions asked in the Introduction about the early manifestations of what would come to be called surgery, its beginnings, and its key figures.

All things change, as Heraclitus noted—some faster than others. We are accustomed to having easy access to convenient, safe, and effective surgical services. You need your gallbladder removed, it's done at your community hospital with no fuss or bother, and you are home the next day. But this scenario is very recent, and far from typical for most of history. When and why did things change and who drove the change?

Surgery developed rapidly over the last two centuries as operative techniques were introduced and improved—but this followed millennia of incremental, minimal activity. It was first essential to have an accurate picture of anatomy (where organs are) and an understanding of physiology (what they do). Religion and society, frequently and ironically, threw up roadblocks to development. Lacking the knowledge of where organs are and what they do, there could be no progress. Once that knowledge was in place, along with related medical capabilities, mainly anesthesia, early surgeons began to develop surgical techniques and actually perform operations. This was the groundwork that led to today's remarkable accomplishments. But before we get to the early chest operations, a useful starting place is with the origins and evolution of surgery itself, including its earliest and crudest manifestations.

The idea that cutting on someone might be good for their health is not intuitively obvious. Perhaps the start was *Homo habilis* (literally, "handy man," one of the earliest species of the genus *Homo,* some two or three million years ago), having had a boil rupture spontaneously or even causing the rupture accidentally after an encounter with a sharp rock, recognizing the salutary value of this serendipity, and repeating it on purpose. Knives chiseled from rocks thought to have been for surgical use have been found dating back to 10,000-8,000 BCE. Skulls from the Neolithic period (some 8,000 years ago) reveal evidence of an apparently popular operation called skull trephination, creating a hole in the cranium by chipping away at the bone with sharpened rocks. One manifestation is a heap of skulls unearthed in South America, each with at least one hole as a result of trephination. Imagine yourself the patient: your scalp is peeled back, and holes in your skull chiseled out with a rock. Even after chewing on the plant of your choice, this had to require remarkable pain tolerance.

This operation was surprisingly widespread, and evidence of its practice has been found across Western Europe, the Levant, and the Americas, especially Peru and Mexico. The purpose of trephination was, presumptively, either to release demons causing headaches or seizures, or to treat skull fractures. This had to be one of the most successful operations ever performed if judged by the low likelihood of the patient returning for a repeat procedure. Actually, some unearthed skulls do have multiple holes from repeat sessions with, presumably, a very persuasive rock-wielder.

The earliest documentation of anything resembling a systematic approach to surgery is found in the Edwin Smith Papyrus. Edwin Smith purchased this insight into Egyptian surgical thought in 1862 in Luxor, but it lay dormant and unread until successfully translated in 1922 by an Egyptologist at the University of Chicago. The

Papyrus was composed around 1500 BCE but is felt to be a copy of an original of some 1500 years prior to that, dating it to approximately 5,000 years ago. This was during the time of Imhotep, considered the father of Egyptian medicine, who kept his opinions free from the spheres of magical and religious thinking. This was in contrast to Asclepius, who, as the father of Western medicine, was considered to be a god gifted with magical powers of healing.

The Papyrus focuses on surgery, especially the surgical approach to traumatized patients. It presents 48 patient scenarios, or cases, of which 27 are about head trauma, and 17 are about chest trauma. The remaining four relate to injuries elsewhere. The document analyzes each case in terms of four categories: the type of injury, the examination of the patient (from which is derived both a diagnosis and prognosis), and, finally, the recommendation for treatment. These recommendations are clearly based on careful examination and observation of the patient, skills still relevant today that many of us worry are being eroded by reliance instead on radiologic imaging techniques such as magnetic resonance imaging, computed tomographic scans, and ultrasound.

In the Papyrus, we also detect adumbrations of today's malpractice concerns: the Papyrus urges physicians not to attempt treatment in those cases when the patient is judged to represent a high risk for a poor outcome. Recommendations of actions physicians should take include suturing of open wounds and splinting of fractures. There is no mention of operating for internal injuries, and in fact, evidence of invasive surgical interventions is sparse; ancient Egyptian mummies are mostly free of scars.

There is no equivalent to the Smith Papyrus in Western medical history. Despite manifestations of interest in and curiosity about human anatomy, progress toward performing significant operative procedures was minimal and erratic. Warriors, as depicted in the Bible and the Iliad, for example, did yank out spears and arrows from wounded comrades and worried over them, but that is about as close as anyone came to performing a surgical procedure for thousands of years of Western history. Substantive surgical development was not seen in the West before we had an accurate understanding of human anatomy, and before the introduction of anesthesia, analgesia, and antisepsis. As discussed below, these were essential for surgeons to be successful, i.e., with patients not only surviving but being improved after an operation.

Galen, a second-century Roman, composed several treatises on anatomy and medical practice which became dogma until well into medieval times. Unfortunately, most of his depictions were simply wrong. For the next millennium, anyone daring to disagree with Galen (or any of the classical authors for that matter) was considered a heretic and found themselves in trouble with both the Church and the medical community. It was impossible to make progress with unreliable and inaccurate underpinnings that couldn't be challenged.

Galen endorsed the teachings of Aristotle that the body was composed of four "humors": blood, phlegm, yellow bile, and black bile. Disease, they both concluded, was a result of an imbalance in one's humors. This led to the practice of "therapeutic" bloodletting which was espoused to restore the appropriate balance. Although the rationale for bloodletting changed over time (the famous Benjamin Rush thought bloodletting reduced harmful tension in blood vessels), the practice continued well into the nineteenth century. Today, of course, we know that losing blood only weakens the body, and not only has no salutary value but can speed the patient's demise. Without bloodletting, in fact, we might have gotten a few more years out of George Washington.

Galen's belief that pus—a noxious, soupy mixture of necrotic tissues, dead and active white blood cells, and bacteria suspended in fluid weeping from inflamed tissues—was not only a good sign but, implausibly, actually necessary for the healing process didn't help either. Galen's misunderstanding gifted us the often-cited oxymoron of "laudable pus," the belief in which resulted in wounds routinely being left with the skin open rather than being sutured closed, essentially guaranteeing infection. On occasion, surgeons even exposed wounds to irritants to induce infection and produce the "laudable" purulent discharge.

Even though he may have seen some internal human anatomy during a stint as physician for gladiators, Galen's published work on human anatomy was based on his dissections of animals. Galen's incorrect descriptions of "human" anatomy lingered in large part because of persistent religious prohibitions against dissection of the "sacred" human body (which is how the trouble began in the first place), and the unchallenged adherence to classical beliefs and teachings. Leonardo da Vinci, along with a few others during the Renaissance, finally began to crack open the door to accurate representations. To satisfy his curiosity and learn for himself the anatomical truth, da Vinci performed cadaver dissections in the first decades of the sixteenth century; however, he (surely self-protectively) kept his precise and accurate drawings and descriptions of his findings in private notebooks which were never shared. He used his observations of internal anatomy as an aid to accurate depictions of his subjects' external appearances in painting and sculpture. (He even noted the need for a stout constitution in performing dissection of a—typically ripe—cadaver by admonishing, "You will perhaps be deterred by the rising of your stomach.")

The Belgian physician Vesalius published in 1545 *De Humani Corporis Fabrica* ("On the Fabric of the Human Body"), which also depicted accurate human anatomy based on actual cadaveric dissections, in contrast to Galen's animal-derived versions. Vesalius' work became the standard text in the West, and finally established a realistic anatomic basis on which to correlate diseases with their organ of involvement, so a target for surgical intervention could at least be envisioned. (The Church's appreciation for Vesalius's contributions took the form of the Inquisition sentencing him to death. The death sentence was eventually commuted to a required pilgrimage to Jerusalem which succeeded in accomplishing the originally desired end, as he died on the return leg of the journey.)

During the Middle Ages, surgeons performed few, if any invasive, (inside a body cavity) surgical operations. There was continued progress in describing human anatomy, partially as a means to speculate about function, i.e., physiology. As religious prohibitions against dissection of humans gave way, dissections became more common, and were performed in amphitheaters for the education of medical students. In the absence of effective preservation, cadaver turnover was brisk and frequent replenishment was necessary. The supply of executed criminals was insufficient to meet demand, which resulted in the new profession of grave robbing by "resurrectionists" who surreptitiously dug up the newly buried and sold the bodies to anatomists.

As all fans of the Broadway musical "Sweeney Todd: The Demon Barber of Fleet Street" know, a limited amount of surgery was practiced by multitaskers called "barber-surgeons" until, in England in 1745, the two professions went their separate ways—leaving behind only the barber pole with its white and red stripes as a reminder of barbering's sanguinary history. Despite the separation, surgeons were still not considered genuine physicians, and rarely attended the era's rudimentary medical schools. (A remnant of that attitude lingers in Great Britain where surgeons are still referred to as "Mister" rather than "Doctor.") An insight into the common regard for surgeons at that time is that Jonathan Swift chose to make Lemuel Gulliver, the ultimate dupe, a surgeon.

These barber-surgeons limited their surgical activity mainly to the infamous bloodletting, amputations, and attempts at nasal reconstruction. (There actually were a surprising number of ways for noses to be lost. Nose amputation was a common form of punishment for criminals; the evidence of the miscreant's deed was as plain as the nose that wasn't on his face. Advanced syphilis took a few, and loss was the price of over-zealous dueling.) A clever technique for reconstruction of the missing part was devised by the Italian Gaspare Tagliacozzi who, in 1597, described his operation of suturing a flap of skin from the patient's arm to his nasal remnant. The surgeon sewed skin, still connected to the patient's left bicep, to the face where the nose had been. Blood vessels took several weeks to grow in from the tissue flap, so it needed to remain connected for several weeks. When the transplanted tissue was sufficiently vascularized to survive without blood supply from the arm, it was severed and "tailored" to resemble a nose as much as possible. Perhaps this punishment incited the common parental admonition to children against sticking their noses in someone else's business.

The closest thing to an operation inside a body cavity was extraction of urinary bladder stones, a common, and quite painful, condition of the times. The surgeon got to the bladder by slicing through the perineum (the part of the body between the genitals and the anus), with the patient positioned on their back, hands tied to feet to expose the target area, and assistants pinning the patient in place. Not every patient survived this brutally painful experience; many succumbed to blood loss and shock. Ephraim McDowell, legendary for being the first to remove an ovarian tumor from a patient, removed bladder stones from the teenaged future President James K. Polk. Polk's recovery allowed him to personify "Manifest Destiny" as his administration pursued the acquisition of what is now the southwestern United States.

There were operations elsewhere in the body. France was a little unsettled in the late seventeenth century as their ruler, Louis XIV, the Sun King, had a problem where the sun didn't shine. He suffered for years from a *fistula*-in-ano, an abnormal connection between the skin and the anus. The rumor it was caused by infrequent bathing and poor hygiene is apparently inaccurate as the king bathed regularly. Charles-Francois Felix, a barber-surgeon, was tapped to treat the fistula. To make sure he was up to the job, Felix was first required to hone his skills through practice on several peasant "volunteers." Fortunately for him, the Sun King recovered uneventfully after his operation. In fact, Felix's success enhanced the reputation of the lowly barber-surgeons: thanks to Felix, they enjoyed an elevation in their status in French society.

Arguably the modern, scientific surgical era was ushered in by the Scotsman John Hunter, whose dominant characteristics were insatiable curiosity, persistence, and stamina. Born in 1728 into a farming household, his education by happy chance anticipated the recommendations set forth several decades later by Rousseau's *Emile*. Rousseau did not emphasize early reading and formal education; he relied upon the innate curiosity of the child to guide their education. Youngsters were to be encouraged to go where curiosity took them, and learning resulted from observation and reflection.

Hunter's development took this prescribed course. He disliked the formality of schools, frequently played hooky, and apparently was never much of a reader. However, he spent his time exploring nature in the Scottish countryside, learning from his own explorations and observations. He also was known for his curiosity as he annoyed family and acquaintances with interminable questions. Such as it was, his formal schooling ended at age 13 and he worked on the family farm until relocating to London at age 20 to live with and work for his older brother William, a surgeon/obstetrician/anatomist with an entrepreneurial bent. William started the first school in England that taught anatomy and dissection (there were medical schools in Scotland, Ireland, and continental Europe but none in England). John was initially required to audition by dissecting a cadaver's arm while his brother looked on. His skill and facility were immediately evident and, as he continued to learn on the job by carrying out his own dissections, he became an instructor in the school, and a successful and very active leader of a band of resurrectionists which served to keep the school well stocked with cadavers.

While teaching anatomy and continuing to supply cadavers for the school, Hunter began a surgical apprenticeship with a noted London surgeon, the standard pathway to becoming an independent practitioner, and the experience distinguishing surgeons from barbers. He also continued to teach anatomy and dissection techniques both with his brother and eventually on his own after the two had a falling out and went their separate ways. Hunter clearly was both an excellent surgeon and teacher of surgical skills; however, as identified by Wendy Moore, he was unique in, "his commitment to founding surgical practice on sound scientific principles." This was consistent with the spirit of the Scottish Enlightenment: looking askance at dogma. He abhorred the lockstep mindset of the times which was to blindly adhere to the ancient and irrational principles promulgated by Aristotle and Galen.

Ironically, he was an empiricist like Aristotle in learning from experience and personal observation, his impulse to categorize what he observed, and questioning received teachings. With his accurate knowledge of anatomy as a foundation, he based his approach to surgical challenges on several factors: common sense, observation, and trial and error experiences with his patients which he supplemented with animal vivisections. An example of his empiricism can be seen in his practice as a military surgeon in the early 1760s during the Seven Years' War with France just after his split from William. He noticed that minimally disturbed gunshot wounds healed faster and more reliably than those treated with the traditional method of vigorous exploration with filthy fingers or forceps to extract the shot.

Over the protestations of colleagues that he was violating classical precepts, he applied this unconventional strategy to the wound care of his patients and must have been gratified to see them do better than those of his peers.

With his military experience behind him, Hunter returned to teaching anatomy and began his independent surgical practice while continuing his experiments to determine best practices and mentoring medical and surgical students until his death in 1793. As his reputation spread and his practice grew, he stopped teaching anatomy to focus on surgery. Over the years, he became a successful and sought-after surgeon both by patients and trainees, although envy diminished his popularity with his surgeon competitors.

He was also not above using himself as an experimental subject: he is thought to have infected himself with gonorrhea, and possibly syphilis, by incising his penis with a contaminated scalpel to investigate how these diseases spread. He likewise encouraged free thinking by his students, unfettered by historical precedent. His revolutionary way of basing the practice of medicine and surgery on experience and observation was spread by his trainees and is now clearly the foundation of the scientific method as applied to surgery. Hunter's ultimate legacy can be found in today's surgeons' respect for the accumulated knowledge while always using experience to increase and modify it. We adhere to Hunter's belief that "surgery should be governed by scientific principles ... based on reasoning, observation, and experimentation," quoting again from Moore.

Hunter was an extraordinary man, albeit quirky, with unlimited stamina and a wide-ranging curiosity about nature that kept him active from his customary rising time of 4:00 a.m. till late at night exploring his many interests which were directly or obliquely related to anatomy or surgery. One of these was in comparative anatomy. At some considerable expense, he obtained the remains of animals, exotic and otherwise, which he carefully dissected, preserving the samples which interested him. To investigate the stages of gestation, he sacrificed animals at intervals following conception and dissected the uterine contents, determining the sequences and patterns of organ development. His notes on this process, not published till after Darwin's bombshell half a century later, make it clear that his analysis of similar anatomic structures in different species resulted in a prescient understanding of the principles of evolution. He manifested an idiosyncratic interest in collecting nature's oddities in humans and animals, displaying his collection in his home and its attached museum. Specimens included the skeleton of a man with gigantism, another of a two-headed cow, and the head of a cockerel onto whose comb he had successfully transplanted the spur from its foot.

One of Hunter's acolytes was the American Philip Syng Physick who brought this legacy home to Philadelphia after studying with Hunter in England. Physick, despite his modest renown, has been tagged, "father of American surgery" because he was the first professor of surgery in the first medical school in America, the University of Pennsylvania. Physick propagated Hunter's precepts and solidified Hunter's reputation in American surgery through his mentoring of individual surgeons, lectures, and publications.

3

RESIDENCY AND RESEARCH

The four years of medical school behind me, I began my training as an intern in the surgery residency program at Hopkins. All trainees—interns and residents—make up what's called the "house staff," the designation coming from the days when all trainees actually resided in the hospital or "house." (In those days, compensation in addition to the living quarters was limited to meals, a uniform, and a minimal stipend.)

Intern: that's what I was. It was demanding: a routine workweek was 100 or more hours in the hospital with only rare days off. Sleep became a valuable commodity; fatigue could not be ignored; often I was on autopilot. I remained happy with my career choice, certain I was in the right place, but exhaustion took a toll.

These were the days when patients were routinely admitted to the hospital a few days before an operation for testing that is now done before admission. They were also kept in the hospital for a week or more following the procedure. This meant surgical wards were always full. As a result, we interns spent more of our time learning and performing patient care duties than developing technical skills in the operating room. Accordingly, I spent the majority of my time outside the operating room tending to patients in the hospital. There was little cross-coverage with other interns, a modern arrangement which allows physicians to keep an eye on each other's patients.

During my time each intern was solely responsible for their patients. This meant I was called if a nurse had a concern, day or night. Unfortunately, as was typical of the era, much of this time and effort was taken up by tasks that contributed little to my training. Like my colleagues I transported patients to get X-rays, started IVs, and arrived well before 6:30 a.m. rounds to draw blood samples for analysis. This was called "scut," work—defined as "routine and often menial labor." The origin of the term is unclear; it may come from the Irish word "scut," designating a person seen as foolish, contempt- ible, or objectionable. In today's teaching hospitals, these tasks are now performed by other hospital personnel, freeing up the house staff for more educational activities.

As an intern, I participated in a limited fashion in operations. When I scrubbed in, I mainly held retractors but did have occasional opportunity to perform minor procedures under supervision. These modest experiences had value, as they helped me get over any perfor- mance anxiety: sharp eyes were watching. Senior surgeons and nurses monitored every move. I was instructed in, and senior surgeons illustrated, proper surgical methodology but no one was reluctant to criticize. Performing these minor operations or the secondary parts of more major ones, such as suturing closed an incision, provided an important opportunity to master essential techniques such as tying square knots, and holding and wielding surgical instruments prop- erly. I was starting to build a framework for advanced surgical skills.

One positive and important result of this immersion was that we interns developed personal responsibility for patients, and an empa- thetic connection to them that superseded all other concerns. I took patients' history and did a physical exam when they were admitted to the hospital, assisted at their operation, and provided daily—and nightly—care until they went home. Recent national modifications by residency supervising agencies have limited the workweek to 80 hours. Better rested residents is a good thing: more opportunity for sleep, study, and home life. Residents now leave the hospital when they have reached their time limit and turn over care of their patients to the "covering" resident.

Yet this tradeoff worries many of us; the potential is a diminished sense of connection between patient and physician; a "shift mentality" is born. Cross-coverage is now common, even for practicing surgeons, not just for house staff. A partner provides care for the patient after I have operated so that I can have a free night or weekend. Although patients are frequently nonplussed when a strange surgeon shows up to care for them after their operation, this practice has never been shown to diminish the quality of patient care or cause poor outcomes. But I worry—as the covering surgeon or resident does not have the same feeling for the patient as the operating surgeon. In addition to this concern, the law of unintended consequences created another change in behavioral patterns. Before the 80-hour limit on the workweek, only a minority of general surgery residents sought more training before entering practice. Now nearly 90 percent of graduating residents obtain an additional year of training as they don't feel sufficiently experienced to act as independent surgeons. We've made the five-year residency less stressful at the cost of adding an additional year of training.

The intern year was challenging but, as a result, I began the second year of training with increased confidence and knowledge. The year of residency after the internship was no less rigorous but daily activities were different. With my peers now called residents, we participated more actively in operations and were generally accorded more responsibility, and even semi-independence on occasion. Embedded in my memory is my first "real" operation, a cholecyst*ectomy* (removal of the gallbladder). After slicing through skin and muscle to expose the gallbladder, I began to cut the surrounding tissue. My chief resident said, softly but with a note of steel: "careful." Undaunted, I continued to nibble at the tissues, a little nervous but mainly exhilarated. As far as I was concerned my career as an operating surgeon had begun. It was during this year, after being exposed to a variety of surgeons and operative procedures, that I recognized I had picked up two interests: thoracic surgery and academic (teaching) surgery.

Where does thoracic surgery fit in the family of surgical special-ties? Thoracic surgery began to be distinguished from general surgery during the early part of the last century as it was realized that expertise in chest operations required further training and a focused dedication after a general surgery residency. Driving this process was an emphasis on the adequacy of the training: doing a sufficient number of chest operations and learning to provide care for the patients. These concerns culminated in the formation of the American Board of Thoracic Surgery in 1948 which assumed responsibility for the quality and sufficiency of training in the specialty, and for certification of individual surgeons. Recently a process has been introduced to assess surgical capabilities and familiarity with new knowledge on an ongoing basis. Just as you would not give someone a permanent driver's license, the initial passage of the examinations for the Boards is no longer a life-time certification. Ironically, physicians initially resisted allowing any organization to have oversight despite the benefit of quality control—losing independence was difficult.

As mentioned in the Introduction, the explosion of coronary artery bypass surgery in the 1970s produced some confusion that lingers. The official designation of my specialty is thoracic surgery. Within are two subspecialties, cardiac surgery and general thoracic surgery for diseases of all else in the chest, most frequently the esophagus and lungs. The designation was born from the association with general surgery and distaste for the previous one: non-cardiac thoracic surgery. No one wants to be identified by what they don't do.

I was drawn to the field of general thoracic surgery. As a resident, I had some interest in general surgery, both its operations and the patients and diseases needing them. However, I experienced more excite-ment and esthetic satisfaction when dealing with chest diseases than with those of the abdominal organs. The techniques of dissection of anatomic structures are similar to those used in performing general surgical procedures but the organs involved and their function, or physiology, I find more interesting and have more appeal. How did these operations come to be? Chapter Four takes us into the early world of chest surgery.

Uncertain how to pursue my nascent interest in the academic aspect of a surgical career, I consulted the Surgery Department chairman at Hopkins and was more or less dispatched after my second residency year to learn about clinical research with the person destined to become my professional mentor, David Skinner, the Chair of the Department of Surgery at the University of Chicago. Mine was a typical pathway into academic surgery. Just as a neophyte surgeon requires training under experienced surgeons to become able to operate safely and independently, research training is indispensable to the eventual ability to be a self-sufficient academician. I did my homework, less straightforward in the pre-Internet era but accomplished through a review of the surgical literature, and arrived in Chicago aware that David Skinner, a thoracic surgeon, was a world authority on the physiology and surgical treatment of diseases of the esophagus.

My research was of the clinical variety, meaning that I carried it out with patients. I addressed clinical questions to add to the understanding of esophageal disorders so that surgical treatment could be improved rather than performing basic science investigations in a laboratory. The first requirement was to increase my familiarity with both the anatomy and physiology of the esophagus. Where is it in the body in relation to other structures and how does it function? Appendix Three reviews these two crucial considerations. Anatomic relationships establish surgical possibilities and limits; there are a finite number of ways a surgeon can modify the esophagus in relation to itself or its neighboring tissues. If a surgeon is unfamiliar with normal esophageal physiology, it is difficult to recognize and characterize deranged and abnormal function, and impossible to develop innovative diagnostic or therapeutic surgical strategies to restore satisfactory performance and relieve symptoms.

Accordingly, before I came to Chicago, I studied anatomy and physiology textbooks, as well as the articles Dr. Skinner had published. Nothing, however, prepared me for the man himself, and the dynamism of his personality. David was a prototypical alpha male, 6'4" tall with broad shoulders, erect posture, and a square chin which, when combined with his black-rimmed glasses, gave him a passing resemblance to Clark Kent. He was a natural leader with no need for pretention. David was equipped with a booming voice. I levitated more than once when he materialized and unleashed behind me. He had a magnetic personality, and it was not long before I knew I wanted to remain at the University of Chicago, and train with him in thoracic surgery.

Skinner, the departmental chairman, and Tom DeMeester, the Chief of the Division of Thoracic Surgery, were renowned general thoracic surgeons and directed my investigations. They shared interests and expertise in the surgical treatment of esophageal disorders. Developing operations to treat and hopefully cure cancer of the esophagus was an ongoing passion but my research activities were focused on what are called "benign diseases." Benign in the medical sense means "not malignant." i.e., not cancerous. It doesn't mean benign in the everyday sense of gentle, kind, or favorable; benign disorders diminish the quality of a patient's life, even if they don't threaten to end it prematurely.

Under the guidance of these two leaders I sought to improve the ability to diagnose and understand diseases of the esophagus that are functional rather than anatomic. Functional disorders impair the ability of the esophagus to perform its normal functions of swallowing and retarding acid reflux, even though it is anatomically normal, i.e., has no tumor, scar tissue, or other structural abnormality. Determining how patients with a functional disorder differed from individuals with normally functioning esophagi provided clues to understanding how the disorder developed, how it might be prevented, and how it might best be treated. One of the two functional disorders of most interest to us was *gastro*esophageal reflux disease (GERD), a condition in which stomach acid refluxes back into the esophagus. Many readers will be all too aware of the heartburn it causes when the acid hits the esophagus. The pharmaceutical companies which manufacture acid suppression drugs in common use inundate the airways with their ads so that GERD, or "acid reflux," is now prominently in the public eye. This was not so in the 1970s.

The other of my research interests was dysmotility conditions of the esophagus: disorders in which the esophagus malfunctions and does not transport food as it should. Either the muscles of the esophagus misfire and fail to push food toward the stomach, or the esophageal sphincters at the top and bottom of the esophagus fail to relax their squeeze to allow food to pass through normally. Both of these breakdowns of the esophagus' food transport mechanism, termed motor or motility disorders, cause a patient to have difficulty swallowing, which we call *dysphagia*.

To evaluate esophageal motility and to quantitate acid reflux, I used specialized catheters that I passed through patients' noses into the esophagus and connected to devices which either detected acid or the function of its muscle. You can imagine the tests were not popular with patients, but the information obtained guided their treatment and added to our understanding of the two entities.

To study dysmotility, I performed a procedure called alternatively "esophageal manometry," or motility. It measures both the pressures being generated by the squeezes along the esophagus which propel food, and by the sphincters at the top and bottom and the pattern of the squeezes; they should progress from top to bottom to propel food. As illustrated in Appendix Three, for this study I threaded a catheter through the patient's nose so that the tip ended in the esophagus. I coated the flexible catheter with a Novocain-like gel—providing lubrication and mild numbing of the tissues—and snaked it gently through the patient's nose so it would curve downward as it encountered the back of the throat where it could be swallowed by the patient and pass down the esophagus.

The catheter had pressure sensors imbedded at varying intervals, enabling me to detect esophageal contractions. I measured the pressures of the contractions and assessed the motility by their pattern. Contractions should be peristaltic: the muscular squeezes should be sequential from top to bottom, so they propel food toward the stomach. If the squeezes are simultaneous, the food bolus is not carried along to its proper destination; it oscillates in the body of the esophagus. In addition, I measured the pressure and relaxation characteristics of the upper and lower esophageal sphincters. After relaxing to allow swallowed food to pass, the upper sphincter, a muscle located at the junction of the pharynx, the back of the throat, and the esophagus, contracts to guard against food regurgitating back into the pharynx where it can be aspirated into the airways. Similarly, the lower sphincter, a muscular complex located where the esophagus and stomach meet, relaxes to allow the swallowed bolus to enter the stomach, afterward contracting to establish a barrier to protect the esophagus from acid reflux. Undergoing this procedure might seem distasteful and, I admit, no patient ever enjoyed the experience sufficiently to ask for a repeat—but most tolerated it without complaint.

The esophageal manometry study was essential for identifying abnormal motility such as when the normal pattern or pressure of contractions was deranged or when there was dysfunction of either sphincter. The prototypical motility abnormality is achalasia, a disorder which causes dysphagia, and difficulty in swallowing. The exam also provided insight into GERD. We were particularly interested in the characteristics of the lower esophageal sphincter (LES) in these patients. How did it contribute to the prevention of acid reflux from the stomach into the esophagus? Why and how did it sometimes fail, and how could a defective LES be surgically restored? Not all questions were definitively answered but two observations were clear. As one might predict, the lower the pressure is in the LES, the more likely reflux will occur. This explains why some foods such as chocolate, alcohol, and coffee cause heartburn—they contain ingredients that reduce the pressure in the LES which diminishes the protection against acid reflux, the cause of heartburn. Swallowed food is not itself the cause of heartburn.

The second characteristic of the LES related to reflux is its length. When it measures to be shorter than the typical length of three to five centimeters reflux is more likely. Overeating and distending the stomach shortens the LES, increasing the likelihood of reflux. Conversely, when most of it is below the diaphragm (and therefore in the positive pressure abdomen rather than the negative pressure chest) the less likely is reflux to occur. These findings also provided clues that defined the important components of a successful anti-reflux operation. Surgeons need operations that raise the pressure or squeeze the LES, and the procedure must anchor the terminal portion of the esophagus within the positive pressure environment of the abdominal cavity. It was not clear that each of the two operative accomplishments was necessary, but both recreated the anatomic relationships that were present in people without acid reflux.

I studied GERD by monitoring acid levels in the esophagus. This examination was the brainchild of Tom DeMeester who shared Skinner's interest in esophageal diseases. DeMeester's goal was to replace (or at least supplement) the subjectivity of what a patient says they feel with objective measurement of the amount of pathological acid refluxed from the stomach into the esophagus. While most patients with GERD have heartburn, it is a sensation detected and reported. It's similar to a person describing pain. Severity is in the mind of the sufferer and people do not feel discomfort the same. An objective measure is a better guide to the severity of the reflux and pH monitoring provides this. This is helpful in confirming a diagnosis and especially important when establishing criteria for surgical intervention.

Typical heartburn is caused by irritation of the esophagus from *gastric* acid refluxing from the stomach. It begins in the upper abdomen and radiates upwards toward the throat, beneath the sternum. As this is roughly the territory of the heart, we can easily understand how "heartburn" acquired its name. However, many people with GERD, despite having enough acid reflux to damage their esophagus, have only mild or occasional heartburn yet may have other symptoms suggesting reflux, such as regurgitation of gastric contents. They may only sense the material rising inside their esophagus, even find the bitter fluid in their mouth, or have a cough caused by aspiration of regurgitated gastric acid into their lungs. The challenge is how to tell if any of these people has severe enough GERD to warrant an operation; or even to be sure that GERD is the correct diagnosis as the other side of the coin is that not all chest pain, even if described by the patient as having a burning component, is actually caused by acid reflux. Angina, the pain caused by diminished blood flow to the heart, can mimic heartburn so there is an important diagnostic role for pH monitoring.

If it is a question of prescribing a medication, a precise diagnosis is less important. If a drug doesn't help, it can simply be stopped.

An operation, however, is permanent and can't be "stopped." If the preoperative diagnosis was incorrect, the patient either lives with outcomes that can range from unhelpful to harmful, or a second and revisional operation are required. From experience I can attest that repeat operations are challenging and less likely to succeed because of scar tissue from the earlier procedure(s). So, both patient and surgeon want any initial operation to succeed, and an accurate diagnosis is an absolute requirement before all operations. An operation to stop reflux won't help heart disease.

For the procedure to measure pH, I placed the tip of the esophageal catheter just above the junction with the stomach, where it had to stay for a full 24 hours. The stomach secretes acid to aid in digestion; as the stomach is by far the most acidic milieu in the body, gastric acid must be the source of any drop in the pH in the esophagus. The catheter in the patient's esophagus detects acid exposure by measuring pH, an exponential measure of acidity. The lower the pH, the greater the acid concentration; moving from a pH of 4 to 3, because it is an exponential measure, identifies a 10-fold increase in the strength of the acid. The catheter was connected to a printer which recorded the pH over the 24-hour period overnight in the hospital.

This once experimental investigation has proved its worth and is now routinely used for patients with or suspected GERD and has brought a welcome ability to objectively measure the amount of acid reflux. The severity of symptoms, especially heartburn, is important as operations are primarily performed to relieve them; having pH monitoring to provide a measure of the amount of acid reflux has been a major advance. The patient acceptance of this test has improved thanks to technological advances. Although the procedure is not painful, to no one's surprise many patients found enduring a catheter through their nose to be unpleasant. The test can now be accomplished with a small acid sensor that is clipped inside the esophagus during an endoscopic procedure. The sensor detects acid reflux and transmits the measured pH level of the acid and the length of time it sits in the esophagus to a data recorder the patient wears on a belt at home. The quite small sensor eventually falls loose from the esophagus and is passed painlessly in a bowel movement. No more catheters through the nose.

My year of clinical research into benign diseases of the esophagus, including GERD but also into disorders of motility, stimulated my interest in treating diseases of the esophagus. I learned the first challenge for the development of new surgical operations for GERD was to understand *pathophysiology*—what went wrong—and shift focus from the anatomic entity of hiatal hernia to the functional abnormality of acid reflux. For the most common dysmotility disorder, achalasia, the first challenge was to define and understand its pathophysiology. What was abnormal about its function? Participating in mapping the abnormalities of the esophagus that resulted in GERD and dysmotility and being exposed to and learning from two leaders of thoracic surgery are what started me on the road to a life in academic thoracic surgery. Consequently, an important goal became securing a position in a thoracic surgery training program after completion of training in general surgery.

We have now begun the story of functional esophageal surgery, i.e., surgery to improve the quality of a patient's life by altering the *function* of an organ—in contrast to an operation to extirpate an anatomical problem—a cancer-containing organ. An analogy: you are considering a new car and spot one you like the looks of. Its "anatomy" is okay—but does it run? That's function.

4

EARLY CHEST SURGERY

The chest and its contents were a mystery to the ancients. It must have stimulated a sense of awe akin to viewing the heavens. As time passed, curious investigators developed an understanding of the function and importance of the heart, lungs, and esophagus. For my colleagues and me the chest is simply our workplace, with no mystery or mystical feelings.

The two operations general thoracic surgeons today most frequently performed are cancer operations: esophagectomy, removal of the esophagus, and excision of part (lobectomy) or all (pneumonectomy) of the lung. But those organs in the recess of the chest were out of reach until very recently. Chest surgeons today routinely perform operations on internal organs, obviously more invasive procedures than pulling out a spear from an impaled victim, draining an abscess, or even bloodletting. Early practitioners of surgical activities, of course, did not distinguish themselves as dedicated to what we would call a specialty. (Today we would call them "hand surgeons"—they operated on anyone they could get their hands on.) Thoracic surgery as a distinct surgical practice is not much older than the past century. The same is true for all surgical specialties.

Chest surgery in the modern sense of operating on the lung, esophagus, and other structures inside the chest requires general anesthesia and endotracheal ventilation. Prior to the late nineteenth century, surgery was limited to care of the aftereffects of wartime chest wounds or accidents, and treatment of chest infections. In essence, after removing spears and arrows, all that the earliest surgeons could do was worry at the side of the victim.

This is not to say worry has gone away; I experienced my share. In common with other surgeons, I spent many hours in intensive care units hoping that adjusting ventilator settings or varying drug dosages would correct a failing patient. But at least I could address the original problem and attempt to help the patient recover from complications. The frustration of worry without the ability to intervene seems intolerable.

Hippocrates suggested, "He who would become a surgeon should join an army and follow it." The influential French surgeon Ambroise Paré in the sixteenth century likewise observed that war is the greatest school of surgery. He felt the battleground was the place to learn about chest injuries and wound care. I'm not sure what could be learned *other* than wound care, as recovery from a penetrating thoracic injury was at that time only a matter of good fortune. Surgeons were limited by a poor understanding of respiratory mechanics, and unprepared to operate inside the chest as is necessary to control active hemorrhage or repair an injured organ. Neither pulling out a spear nor suturing a skin laceration constitute definitive care.

What early surgeons were able to do was suture closed lacerations of the skin and muscles of the chest wall which did not penetrate the rib cage. The injuries healed more rapidly than if they had been left open. Closure also prevented bacteria from getting into the muscle below the skin and setting up an infection. Injuries penetrating to the inside of the chest challenged the early surgeon, as they were potentially lethal. There was both uncertainty and controversy at the time regarding the treatment of these penetrating injuries which had the potential to wreak havoc with any combination of the heart, lungs, and aorta. Paré was one of the first to try treating wounds in the thoracic cavity. His initial profession, preparing him for delicate surgical undertakings, was as a blacksmith.

Paré's humility and religious convictions are captured by his famous statement about one of his patients, *"Je le pansai, Dieu le guérit."* ("I bandaged him, God cured him.") Paré, however, erred in advising surgeons not to suture closed penetrating wounds. He recommended leaving them open, although he worried about the entry of cold air into the chest doing damage to the heart. There was actually a theoretical, modest benefit to not closing the tissues in the setting of a wound penetrating through the rib cage: blood could drain out of the open chest rather than accumulate inside where it would compress the lung. However, this communication between the chest cavity and the atmosphere compromised the patient's ability to breathe, as the lung on the injured side collapsed since the chest could not generate the negative pressure necessary to maintain inflation.

Historically, we see early surgeons picking up on sporadic clues that a closed chest was better for breathing. Baron Larrey, surgeon to Napoleon's army, sewed up one soldier's chest wound while the injured man struggled to breathe, and noted, "The wound was scarcely closed, when he breathed freely and felt easier." Restoring the integrity of the chest wall protected the lung from being collapsed by the pressure of atmospheric air. (The lung has the consistency of a wet sponge; it has no rigid support. It is held in an expanded state by a vacuum created by negative pressure inside the chest. If the chest is open to the outside, the vacuum is lost, the lung collapses and cannot function.) Unfortunately, the lesson from this was not generally appreciated; closure of open chest wounds did not become standard practice until World War I. Upon consideration, that's not so surprising: in the absence of medical journals and surgical society gatherings (much less the Internet), surgeons had no reliable way to disseminate news of new techniques or information.

I am impressed by Larrey's insights; he was ahead of his time in many ways. He invented the ambulance, which he originally used to convey the surgeon and his instruments onto the battlefield to care for the wounded—of the enemy as well as the French. His colleagues eventually began to use ambulances to transport wounded soldiers to field hospitals. Both strategies gave French soldiers at least a chance for survival, in contrast to being left to lie, suffer, and almost certainly die where they fell.

It's hard not to smile when movies or television dramas portray a wild west hero urgently extracting a bullet from a wounded comrade. Not always necessary; sometimes a bad idea. Bullets fired from guns are, in fact, at least partially sterilized by the heat generated as they pass through the air. It is true, of course, that bacteria infest clothing or other material bullets pick up from the patient. "Foreign bodies," as they are called by surgeons, in combination with badly traumatized tissue (such as muscle that has been deprived of its blood supply and is becoming necrotic) can be a source of future infection. A surgeon should remove safely accessible bullets and these foreign bodies from the wound, and excise all the tissue that is not viable, a process called "*debridement*." But retrieving bullets buried in deep tissues can be more trouble than it's worth to both surgeon and patient. The search can disrupt and traumatize uninjured organs and, unless in a threatening location, such as near a pulsating blood vessel which can be eroded, can safely be left where they lodged. Lead poisoning can result eventually as lead is leached from a bullet, but initial conservatism is still appropriate.

This was not understood until recently; in the past, surgeons frequently fixated on retrieving musket balls and other penetrating objects from victims' chests. Hochberg tells of an injured Colonel in Spain in 1815 who 'procured the aid of a surgeon [who] ... proceeded to probe and dilate [his chest wound] until the Colonel, losing patience, asked him what he was looking for. "The ball, to be sure," replied the surgeon. The Colonel's reply was brief: "Why did you not tell me that sooner; the ball is in my waistcoat pocket."'

This preoccupation, coupled with the American surgeons' lack of appreciation of the germ theory, produced a perfect surgical storm which was fatal for President James Garfield in 1881. An assassin shot him, and Garfield was immediately taken to the White House for care (a comment on the confidence in hospitals). There he fell into the clutches of the infelicitously named Dr. Bliss, who spent the summer probing and exploring the wound with bare, unwashed hands in an unsterile environment searching for a bullet that was nestled in fatty tissue and causing no harm. The inevitable infection finally killed Garfield the following September.

When did chest operations other than removal of spears and bullets and suturing of lacerations begin? Lung operations, removing all (pneumonectomy) or part (lobectomy), for cancer are routine today. I performed them on a regular basis. Lung operations began when surgeons carried out—very limited—procedures when they had to deal with patients whose injuries to the chest resulted in part of a lung protruding outside the chest. Before this trauma experience no one had considered removing part of the lung. The first operation we know of was in 1499 when an Italian surgeon "resected" a portion of lung. His contribution really amounted to no more than scraping away necrotic tissue from a lung which had partially herniated through a chest wound. Even this minimal surgery was probably unnecessary: compression by the ribs on the herniated lung would have been sufficient to cut off its blood supply, meaning it would simply eventually become necrotic, slough off, and fall away from the patient. His encounter was, however, enough to encourage other surgeons to see the possibility. These early surgeons gained experience and set the stage for human lung operations by trying them in animals.

In addition to these uncommon scenarios, surgeons were most often able to help when there was an infection in the chest. Now, of course, the mainstay for treatment for most bacterial infections is the appropriate antibiotics. But before antibiotics became available, surgery was the only available therapeutic option. Even today, there are occasions when surgical drainage of a purulent collection, or removal of infected tissue, must be added to the antibiotic regimen to achieve complete control of an infection.

These early surgeons were involved with patients with four kinds of chest infections, found either in the lung or the pleural space. The first was lethal tuberculosis (TB) which primarily attacks the lungs. Emphasizing its lethality, in the USA it was called "consumption" because it consumed the sufferer. This common infection was a scourge and decimated populations before effective drug therapy in the twentieth century. Yet most people exposed to the TB bacillus by breathing it in never develop an infection. When it takes hold, however, the infection is remarkably destructive. The bacteria destroy enough tissue that they can hollow out a cavity in the lung.

The cavities harbor TB but are usually empty otherwise. On occasion, bacteria or even fungus migrate from the bronchial system and move in. When this happened surgeons first attempted to drain the infected material from these cavities. A better strategy was to actually obliterate the cavities. The TB bacillus could not survive if there were no cavity. Without a cavity, the bacilli could not create a reservoir of bacilli which the patient could cough up to infect others, a significant public health threat. Also, the cavities put the person at risk for serious, even exsanguinating, hemorrhage. The TB bacteria destroy the lung substance but not the hardier blood vessels which traverse the cavity. When these blood vessels are no longer protected by surrounding lung tissue, they are easily torn when the infected person coughs. There is also the possibility of erosion of arteries by the TB bacillus or other bacterial organisms in the cavity. Either way, massive bleeding can occur.

Beginning in the late nineteenth century and continuing through the first half of the twentieth, surgeons adopted the obliteration strategy and began deliberately collapsing the infected lung, addressing the problem directly. Collapse therapy was based on several considerations. The TB bacillus is aerobic, which means it requires oxygen to survive. (This is why it gravitates to the lungs.). Collapsing a lung deprives TB of air and oxygen. In addition, surgeons felt that cavities would have a better chance to heal if the lung was at rest and compressed so that the cavities were allowed to fall in upon themselves and be obliterated by the sides healing to each other.

There were several ways to accomplish collapse. One of the first was to use a syringe to instill air into the pleural cavity (inside the chest but outside the lung) which squeezed the lung down. Alternatively, surgeons made a small chest incision to allow air to enter the chest; with no more negative pleural pressure, the lung's elastic tissue contracted, and the lung collapsed. The presumption, usually correct, was that the patient could live with only the other lung functioning. Another collapse method was to target the phrenic nerve which activates the diaphragm. The surgeon can find the nerve where it traverses the neck so it's not necessary to enter the chest. A phrenicotomy, cutting the phrenic nerve on one side, did the job. Alternatively, the surgeon crushed the nerve with a surgical clamp. (Crushing gave the nerve the opportunity to heal and recover function over several months.) Either way, the diaphragm was paralyzed and could no longer descend normally. As the diaphragm rose it compressed the infected lung, squeezing the cavity while leaving the patient's other lung to function normally and sustain the patient.

Over the years new methods were introduced. Plombage (packing the pleural space—between the lung and the inner chest wall—with a foreign substance, e.g., wax or Lucite balls, to compress the lung), and thoraco*plasty* (removing several ribs so that the muscles and other tissues of the chest wall would fall inward) are both effective. All these procedures either exerted pressure on and compressed the lung or allowed the lung to collapse on itself, thus bringing the walls of the cavity into contact with each other. After the collapse intervention, patients recovered in hospitals or were placed in a sanitorium. Though the results of lung collapse are not well documented, it is clear that many patients did improve. Until the advent of efficacious antibiotics, collapse therapy supplemented by rest and good nutrition was the main treatment of TB, especially when lung cavities complicated the situation.

The advent of effective drugs to treat TB resulted in a marked decrease in its incidence. Unfortunately, there has been a resurgence of tubercular infection due in large part to diseases such as AIDS which suppress the immune system and impair its ability to fight off infection. Also, malnutrition, common among drug users, weakens their immune capability. Although efficacious drugs are available to treat patients, some have persistent disease or develop cavitary complications, either because their treatment began too late, or their TB organisms are resistant to even combinations of the drugs. Surgery is frequently necessary in these instances. For contemporary patients, an operation is most frequently indicated for persistent infection, cavities complicated by bacterial or fungal superinfection, or a history of bleeding. When an operation is needed, collapse therapy has been replaced by a more direct surgery. The surgeon removes the infected lung lobe—and the cavity it harbors.

This is tricky surgery, technically more challenging than a

lobectomy for lung cancer because of the intense inflammatory reaction to the infection. The lung's central, connecting hilar structures are buried in an inflammatory mass which obliterates normal tissue planes separating anatomic structures. The inflammation and infection weld together blood vessels and lung tissues that are normally easily dissected apart. Consequently, it's difficult to distinguish anatomic features and a vigorous tug by the surgeon on one part of the lung can easily tear a hole in a blood vessel, with the obvious potential consequences of shock or even death due to blood loss. Operations on these patients are done by experienced thoracic surgeons with the patience and expertise to perform these painstaking procedures.

A cavity in the lung with bacteria is a form of an abscess and TB can cause this, but TB is not the only culprit. A lung abscess can also be a result of bacterial pneumonia which does not, or only insufficiently, responds to the usually effective antibiotics. Less frequently, an abscess can also result from bacteria spilling into the lung after aspiration of gastric contents. This can happen when someone vomits when their sensorium is compromised by alcohol or drugs which suppress the normal, protective cough reflex. Before ventilators and anesthesia came along which permitted, as I'll explain below, operating on the lung inside the chest, the goal of surgical treatment of lung abscesses was to cut into the patient's chest at the site of the presumed abscess, hopefully located by examination of the patient. Then it was necessary to cut and probe through the chest wall to enter the abscess cavity to provide the purulent contents a way to drain out. Even in the era of antibiotics, the primary principle of treating any abscess in any part of the body is to cut it open and create a passage through the skin to the outside so the purulent material can drain out. The abscess cavity can then heal from the inside out. This is called establishing external drainage and was the goal of the early chest surgeons.

What exactly is an abscess? It is a collection of pus, a liquid. It is more like a pond than a river. As a pond is surrounded by land, an abscess is contained by surrounding tissue. A stagnant pond is neither fed nor drained by a stream; similarly, an abscess is not connected to blood vessels. If antibiotics cannot get inside an

abscess, antibiotic drugs have no access to the bacteria and are ineffective. This explains why drainage is essential and antibiotics alone
are inadequate. There is another reason. Barry Wood, one of my
medical school professors and a former All-American quarterback at
Harvard (in the era before big money was available to tempt him into
a professional football career) discovered that bacteria in the core of
an abscess are quiescent—like the center of a pond—and therefore
unharmed by antibiotics which require bacterial metabolic activity
to be effective.

Precisely locating the chest incision was important for the early
surgeon's intent on draining a lung abscess: the infection induces
an inflammatory reaction that creates adhesions, a form of scarring,
that stick the lung to the chest wall. The surgeon's incision at this
point enters into the abscess cavity; the lung cannot collapse because
inflammation has tethered it to the chest. If the surgeon cuts into
the thorax in the wrong location he does not hit the cavity, but he
does allow air to enter the pleural cavity through the incision; the
lung collapses, the patient struggles to breathe, and the abscess is not
drained. Today's surgeons use chest x-rays to localize the abscess,
improving the odds of finding the precise location of the infection. (In
fact, now when drainage is required most lung abscesses are treated
by radiologists who, using CT scan guidance, place a tube through
the skin into the cavity.) Today, we infrequently encounter lung
abscesses, and even when found they rarely require surgical intervention. Our (usually) effective drugs to treat TB have reduced the
incidence of tubercular cavities. Early antibiotic treatment of pneumonia diminishes the likelihood of abscess development. Even when
an abscess complicates pneumonia, most patients can be successfully
treated with antibiotics as the abscess can drain into a *bronchus*,
be coughed up, and spat out. This process is neither pleasant nor
elegant, but it's effective and spares patients an operation.

The least common chest infection early surgeons faced was
bronchiectasis, a variant of pneumonia. I mention this in passing
as operations for this infection were not possible in early times.
Bronchiectasis is an infection of the airways, the bronchi, which
has eroded their supporting framework. The affected and weakened
bronchus becomes permanently dilated (the meaning of the suffix

"-ectasis") and forms a pool of bacteria and pus which, because of the damaged bronchus, can't be coughed up and cleared. As with lung abscesses, this condition is much less common today: physicians can initiate effective antibiotic therapy early in the course of a pneumonia to eradicate the bacteria. Bronchiectasis was more frequently encountered in the nineteenth century. Removal of the diseased lung is the only surgical treatment, which became possible late in the century at the same time as thoracotomy became realistic. I'll say more about this in the chapter focusing on lung surgery.

The final chest infection early surgeons struggled with was in the chest but not in the lung; rather, it was in the pleural space, inside the chest but outside the lung. Under normal conditions, the lungs fully occupy the chest cavities; however, they are only attached centrally, where what is called the *hilum* shelters blood vessels to and from the heart and lungs and the main bronchi from the *trachea* (windpipe). It is, therefore, possible for air or fluid to accumulate between the lung and the chest wall—in the pleural space—and compress the relatively insubstantial lung. (This makes possible the collapse therapy for TB.) When uninfected fluid accumulates in the chest cavity, we call it a pleural effusion.

An infected pleural fluid collection is called "empyema," and it is equivalent to an abscess in the chest. Empyema is most frequently a complication of pneumonia; it is the result of the bacteria migrating from the infected lung into the chest cavity. It can also result from a penetrating chest injury that brings bacteria into the pleural space. (So, it can complicate a chest operation.) Where exactly the infection was in the chest was not easy to answer before x-ray guidance, but could be suspected on clinical grounds, such as where the patient felt the worst pain.

As for all abscesses, external drainage of the purulent contents is required. The famed Hippocrates, one of the fathers of Western medicine, performed the first recorded instance of chest drainage for empyema. He cut between two ribs and then cleverly packed the incision with cloth which allowed the infected pleural fluid to drain out but prevented air from entering the chest. We have only a few other historical examples of surgical drainage; surgeons were most successful when the infection had advanced enough to burrow between two ribs, and present to the surgeon a red, swollen target like a large boil just beneath the skin. This condition, termed "empyema necessitans," ensured that the surgeon's incision would enter the infected space with little risk of damaging the underlying lung. In the late eighteenth century, the influential British barber-surgeon Samuel Sharp, true to his name, reinvigorated interest in surgical drainage by providing directions for surgeons planning a small thoracotomy to evacuate the infected material of an empyema. As was the case with lung abscesses, x-ray capability arrived a century later to provide the ability to both make a definite diagnosis and guide the surgeon.

In the absence of knowledge, some well-intended surgical forays were both quirky and amusing. When planning to drain an empyema, the surgeon ran up against an ongoing controversy regarding the effect of air entering the pleural cavity. One surgeon in 1867 was so convinced that air alone could induce a lethal infection that he submerged patients under water for his operations. Hochberg, seeing the humor, wrote, "One can imagine the surgeon dressed in boots and coverall carrying a sac of instruments in one hand and a pair of swimming wings in the other as he approaches the patient who is sitting in a bathtub full of water." This is just more evidence of how poorly the so-called "germ theory" was understood. Drainage of the empyema by insertion of a percutaneous chest tube (through the skin and into the pleural space) in combination with antibiotics, is today the standard approach and frequently sufficient treatment. This common procedure today is performed at the bedside using local anesthesia.

When inserting a chest tube, I infiltrated the skin and deeper tissues with a local anesthetic, but even so, it caused some pain and was uncomfortable until removed. Yet tube drainage usually spared the patient an operation. When the infection has gone untreated long enough to fester and form multiple pockets of pus, one or even two chest tubes are insufficient to drain all of them; an operation becomes necessary. The goal of the operation is to fully evacuate the infected contents and make sure the lung can completely expand so there is no longer a space between lung and chest wall. In my early days, this required an open thoracotomy, teasing the infected material from the lung and chest wall and scooping it out with my gloved hands. Now the operation can now usually be performed using minimally invasive techniques with small incisions, a video camera, and instruments long enough to reach all areas inside the chest, equally effective and less stressful for the patient.

Having caused, witnessed, and treated the pain my patients suffered after I cracked their chest, it continues to amaze me that patients of yesteryear were able to tolerate these kinds of invasive thoracic surgical interventions. All procedures involved cutting and probing of chest tissues with minimal or no anesthesia during their performance or analgesia afterward during the period of convalescence. Multiple factors contributed to patient stoicism. In contrast to us, they were living in an age without analgesic medication to relieve even the many and common quotidian aches and pains to which our flesh is heir, much less narcotics for occasional severe pain. So, their tolerance level for pain, whether inherent or acquired, was built up from experience. (On the other hand, there were, until recently, no prescription opiates to lead to addiction, a major problem at present.) They had no choice; tolerating pain was the price of living. Suffering resulting from an abscess or pus brewing inside the chest would be an incentive to submit to the surgeon's knife, painful as it might be. And a patient intolerant of the surgeon's painful interventions simply did not survive their infection.

5

COMPLETION OF
RESIDENCY

After I finished my year of research, I moved on into the general surgery residency at the University of Chicago. The research experience taught me how to think critically and structure clinical investigations. I knew it was what I needed for a foundation in academia but was energized to return to the clinical world. Completing general surgery training was important, but my eye was on my ultimate goal of the thoracic surgery residency. Surgeons operate. As a more senior resident, I more frequently was the operating surgeon, always under supervision. I acknowledged the value of learning all aspects of patient care in the initial years, but no longer limited to just assisting or performing minor operations, I was eager to learn to carry out major operative procedures.

The Chicago faculty were surgeons with international stature, and enviable role models for residents. Like their peers around the country, they were of the generation schooled to believe in the curative value of "big" operations for cancer that removed much more than the affected organ. The logic went as follows: removing the organ, with its cancer, inside an envelope of a substantial amount of surrounding tissue, especially the regional lymph nodes that might contain cancer cells that had the potential to spread to distant parts of the body, would increase the likelihood that all malignant cells had been captured by the surgery. This generation of surgeons believed such extensive operations were necessary for an actual cure of the cancer. This dogma has since been challenged and even disproved for some malignancies such as breast cancer.

There was some justification for this aggressiveness—at that time the chemotherapy larder was not as well stocked as it is today, neither in quantity nor efficaciousness, and immunotherapy was not on the scene. For many cancers and many patients, an aggressive operation was the sole hope for complete cure. Even today, the type of extensive operation described above is associated with improved patient survival for some malignancies. However, although inspired by good intentions, many of these operations for cancer which sweep up wide swathes of tissue are both unnecessary and associated with excessive morbidity. They stress the patient as they take longer to perform and are accompanied by the loss of more blood as the dissections range into surrounding structures. I cared for many patients whose unnecessarily aggressive procedures brought complications such as enormous swelling of the arm after radical mastectomy for breast cancer or landed them in the intensive care unit; some not to survive.

I was taught during my residency to perform a radical mastectomy for breast cancer (although as a thoracic surgeon, I never operated for breast cancer afterward). This is a rarely performed operation today. Here is why: the surgeon performing a radical mastectomy removes not only the entire breast, but also several muscles of the chest wall, and all the lymph nodes in the *axilla* (armpit). Nowadays, the surgeon resects only the part of the breast with the tumor (inelegantly called a "lumpectomy"), but no muscle and only selected lymph nodes. Coupled with radiation therapy, chemotherapy, and immunotherapy, this modern approach produces the same therapeutic outcomes and cure rates, without the pain and disfigurement that accompanied radical mastectomy.

While I certainly don't long for the good old days, the challenge of learning to safely perform technically complex operations such as the radical mastectomy helped me develop skills for the operating room. Each surgeon taught us their preferred operative techniques.

The differences included the location of the skin incision, which tissues to dissect first, how much tissue to remove, and which instruments to use for grasping or holding tissues. Most differences were unimportant and, though strongly believed in, only reflected personal preference. I benefited from the exposure to a variety of surgical approaches by incorporating components from each teacher into my final operative style.

I was given significant responsibility for patient care. As a chief resident, I organized my team of junior residents, made rounds twice a day with them and students, and reported to the attending surgeon who might accompany the team or make his own rounds. I was often the operating surgeon. I was still supervised by the faculty surgeon during most operations but on occasion allowed to operate independently when the attending surgeon had seen enough to trust. As "chiefs," we were expected to be leaders of the residency program and, in turn, teachers of junior residents. I remembered my neophyte years and tried to pass on what I had learned about patient care and the performance of operations.

A common aphorism for learning operative techniques was "see one, do one, teach one." The idea, supported by pedagogical theory, is that becoming able to teach—that is, to lead a junior resident through an operation—makes clear you have mastered the procedure. As the teacher, it is necessary to orchestrate the activity; it's far more challenging than being the learner and responding to direction. An analogy is driving to a new destination and being directed by your companion who directs you left or right. You arrive safely but not necessarily able to repeat the drive on your own, as you didn't pay attention to street names. Confidence in your mastery of the knowledge of the route comes when you are able to switch places and direct someone else.

But, as you would expect, it wasn't that cut and dried for complex major procedures; a resident might have to see some operations several times and perform increasingly more of its components before finally being able to carry it out from start to finish. The progression from seeing to doing to teaching identifies the necessary evolution from theoretical understanding to acquiring technical adequacy to being sufficiently competent to lead a less experienced resident through an operation. A better aphorism for mastering surgery would be "see some, do some, teach some." I was on both ends as I aged through residency. The first time I was allowed the position of the operating surgeon and simply told to get started with no further instructions, it became clear that I had not really mastered all the elements: where to place the instruments to provide exposure of the operative field, which tissue should be initially incised, and other considerations. In my previous operations, the senior resident or attending surgeon had directed and I had complied; I needed to learn the street names.

This incremental process was repeated four times during my year as a chief resident; the four chief residents rotated to spend three months on each of the four clinical services. Each service had its coterie of surgeons who had specific interests. The surgeons on one service, for example, performed the majority of the department's breast and endocrine surgery. Another mainly performed kidney transplantation; no other organs were being transplanted at that time. A third service focused on patients needing operations on their liver, gallbladder, or pancreas. The surgeons of the final of the four specialized in colorectal surgery. We residents in our final year of training developed operative/technical competence through many hours in the operating room. The attending surgeons still kept a close eye and were on hand when we encountered a challenge or new finding, but I was given an opportunity to deal with the situation first.

I solidified my decision-making and leadership skills during this ultimate year. There was a team of residents on each service, and I shepherded my team of junior residents and medical students—and learned to judge on both whom and when to operate. A patient may urgently need an operation, but time is well spent making sure they are in the best possible condition to tolerate the procedure. Needless delay is harmful but, for example, investing a few hours giving intravenous fluids to a dehydrated patient needing an operation for blockage of the intestines is to the patient's benefit; they are fitter and in better shape to tolerate an operation. Surgeons are not famous for their patience but sometimes it is called for.

Equally important was learning to use judgment to decide on whom *not* to operate. There is frequently considerable pressure exerted by family members and referring physicians to do "all you can" because it's the patient's "last hope." This pitch resonates with the typically aggressive surgeon. Unfortunately, there are situations from which a patient cannot be rescued, either because of their inability to endure the stress of a major operation or a cancer sufficiently widespread that cure is not possible. Submitting these patients to an operation they have no realistic hope of surviving or benefitting from simply prolongs suffering for both patient and family. It is hard to say "no," but is much kinder for patients and families than performing a futile operation and inflicting more pain and suffering. This was a hard lesson for me to learn, as my instinct also was to persevere. It took standing at a bedside in an Intensive Care Unit with a grieving family, watching as my patient, plugged into IVs and catheters and on a ventilator, inexorably dwindled after my futile operation, for the lesson to sink in. I had operated on the patient's cancer of the esophagus but had been unable to remove all the lymph nodes harboring metastases. He was doomed and likely to spend most of his remaining days in the hospital. There is neither dignity nor benefit to being heroic in a hopeless situation.

Each resident team on a service remained together for a month or two. We became very close and reliant on each other. There was much to do: perform operations, check patients' wounds, evaluate new fevers, start IVs, perform histories and physical exams on patients being admitted, review new X-rays, and the list went on. We made rounds in the morning before starting operations and generated our scut list of tasks to be taken care of. We worked together, helped each other out, and real friendships blossomed.

Ultimately, I reached the end of my general surgery training and went directly into the two-year thoracic surgery residency which included training in both general thoracic surgery with Drs. Skinner and DeMeester, and cardiac surgery. Though it was not my main interest, my participation in cardiac surgery was positive, thanks to the effervescence and teaching skills of the senior surgeon, an affable man of Greek descent with a mercurial temperament. "Avuncular" is an appropriate descriptor if your uncle is intermittently turbo-charged. His passion and enthusiasm were contagious, although his unpredictability was disconcerting. His idiosyncratic, irreverent manner put off some of his peers and prevented an ascent into national academic stardom, but he was a superb teacher of surgical technique due to his patience with the residents and his own dexterity.

Despite my enjoyment of my time with him, I was not moved to consider a career in cardiac surgery. I must admit that there is a visceral thrill when operating on the heart. It is also a humbling feeling to hold a human heart in your hands; however, this diminished after many experiences. Coronary artery bypass grafting was by far the most common heart operation at this time. There is a technical challenge to create a meticulous *anastomosis*, the sewing of either a vein or artery to the obstructed coronary artery supplying blood to the heart's muscle. However, I found the operation repetitious. I was not attracted to replicating this operation on a daily basis and maintained my commitment to general thoracic surgery. As it turns out, coronary bypass is now less frequently performed, thanks to the introduction of stenting performed by cardiologists. There is a greater variety of cardiac operations now than when I trained but they weren't available to tempt me during residency.

Yet as a future thoracic surgeon, I benefited in several ways from the experience of operating on the heart and aorta. One of the most valuable was developing gentleness with organs and precision with surgical technique so that I was comfortable dealing with blood vessels, especially those that are diseased and fragile. This asset was quite useful in later years when operating for trauma and on the lung's arteries and veins. Also, I learned to remain calm and prepared to cope with torrential bleeding when something went awry, an occupational hazard when dealing with the heart and its great vessels; not a time to panic.

When removing a lung, for example, it is necessary to divide major arteries. Clamps can slip off a blood vessel and tears happen when cutting into or dissecting tissue. I have experienced my share of these mishaps. The result is a pool of blood quickly obscuring the surgical field making it difficult to see and control the offending leak. Haste in restoring control is essential but calm, not frenzied, actions are called for so that the situation is not made worse. The surgeon must quickly compress the miscreant vessel to stop the bleeding and find a way to place a clamp so the operation can proceed.

The general thoracic service was always busy, exposing me to an extensive variety of patients and an array of operative experiences. Skinner had an international reputation and was frequently referred patients for treatment of benign or malignant esophageal disease. DeMeester was earlier in his career but also a well-established surgeon with a busy practice. As mentioned previously, Belsey himself spent several months in Chicago each year. Mr. Belsey (British remember) was of average height, stocky with the ruddy complexion of an outdoorsman, and capped by swept-back silver hair. He didn't have Skinner's imposing height or booming voice but radiated a quieter charismatic presence that generated respect. He frequently made rounds with my resident team as we walked through the hospital. His insights were always instructive; he was knowledgeable, but there was more. His "feel" for patients and operations was remarkable. He and Skinner on the left are shown in Figure 2 in the operating theater of the University of Chicago circa 1980; two alpha males at ease in their domain.

Each of the three had his own teaching style and all were superb surgeons. Dr. Skinner was in and out of the operating room supervising, always knowing when to personally step in, but, as the department chair, he was encumbered with administrative duties that competed for his time. Mr. Belsey frequently scrubbed into these operations and guided me through them. He had a rare talent for navigating between speed and gentleness, the Scylla and Charybdis of surgical technique. A lengthy operation means a patient is under general anesthesia for a prolonged time and body cavities are open and exposed to possible bacterial contamination—not good for the patient. Yet, it is possible to become so worried about time passing that the surgeon rushes an operation. (There is even the "gunslinger" mentality which urges some surgeons to out-race their peers.) An undue preoccupation with haste can be rough on internal tissues as they are tugged aside during surgery; injuries to them can result.

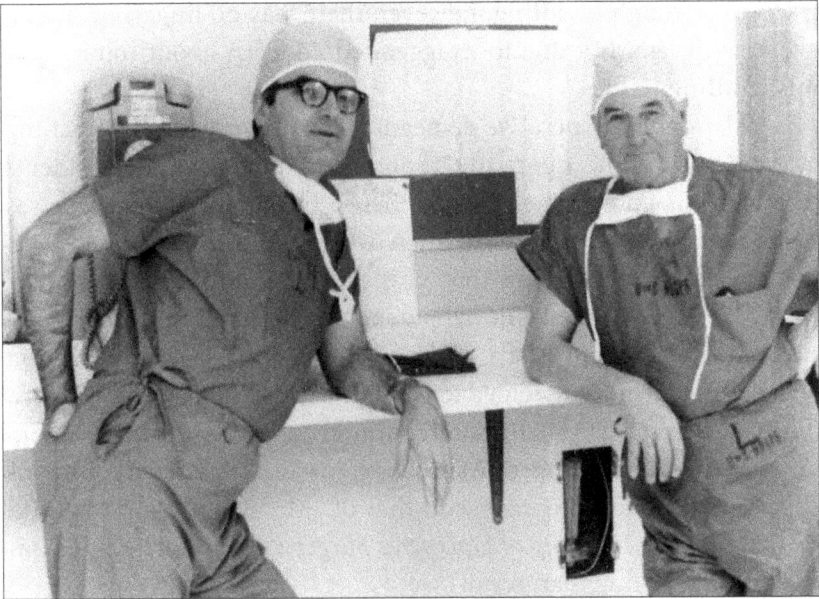

FIGURE 2

These iatrogenic injuries can, of course, increase complications of the operation. A tear in the spleen can be the result of tugging on the stomach which is connected by several blood vessels; the spleen then must be removed. Imprecise suture placement can lead to a devastating breakdown of an anastomosis of the esophagus to the stomach following esophagectomy.

Belsey personified the ideal balance. He was calm and methodical in his operative technique but not plodding. His operations moved along because there was no wasted motion. I loved watching Belsey quickly identify the correct tissues to dissect which would separate organs and release them from their attachments within the body. He never interrupted his progress with hesitation. He had an algorithm—a plan for the sequence of operative maneuvers—for each procedure and calmly proceeded from A to B to C. I saw that his hands moved with purpose and that it was because of this, not speed, that his operations were expeditious. Yes, his surgeries progressed at a reasonable pace, but I also saw that patients' tissues were manipulated gently, and with respect. Nothing was traumatized by excess traction or rough handling; however, there was no lingering, as can occur with timidity due to exaggerated concern about injuring or mishandling tissues.

Belsey's calm operative demeanor was mirrored in his teaching of residents in the operating room. He challenged the residents to match his commitment to excellence but at the same time was encouraging and supportive when we fell short. He never belittled the learner, believing that only eroded confidence and interfered with the resident's development. I have observed other good surgical teachers, but I have also seen those who used intimidation on a regular basis and seemed to take pleasure in harassing residents. (Such bullying was much more common in earlier years; I seldom see or hear of it any longer.) At any rate, few teachers had a conscious educational philosophy to match that of "Mr. B." In his thoughtful treatise *On the Teaching of Operative Surgery*, he set forth an unimpeachable teaching manifesto:

> "It may be possible to teach the principles of a surgical procedure by a written or illustrated description but not the subtleties of operative technique.... The trainee is ... literally in the hands of his instructor whose first responsibility is to demonstrate the basic principles of good operative technique: decision, deliberate planned manoeuvres, gentleness, clean cutting and no rough handling of tissues.... There must be no haste but no purposeless time-wasting activity. Speed in operating should be an achievement and not an objective.... Of supreme importance is the demonstration of that fundamental virtue of the good surgeon: equanimity, and the ability to deal calmly with any untoward event during the procedure."

Belsey meant and lived by these precepts.

It was also true that Mr. Belsey did not suffer fools easily. These were easily identified as surgeons holding opinions different from his. A particular *bête noire* was surgeons who touted the results of a new operation they devised without waiting to see if the results held for the long term. Since his surgical instincts were invariably correct,

I never saw this trait as a problem. He really was not arrogant, just uninterested in social pretense. This behavior did affect him, however. His directness and willingness to give public criticisms of his peers at surgical meetings, although delivered in a mellifluous British accent, ruffled enough feathers to prevent his being knighted, an honor accorded to several British surgeons of his era. I consider this unfortunate; his contributions to surgery were commensurate with those who were so honored. And I must add that self-confidence is not hard to find in thoracic surgeons; I have never known a surgeon who, like the children of Garrison Keillor's town in *Prairie Home Companion*, wasn't certain he or she was above average.

6

ANESTHESIA AND VENTILATION

With the advent of anesthesia and ventilation, surgery emerged from the restrictive era of unchallenged adherence to classical dogma, and surgeons began to operate (with variable success) for chest injuries and infections. But there were limits to what they could do. Patients could tolerate only so much pain and to perform precise operations; surgeons required a still patient, so anesthesia was needed. Additionally, for chest operations there was the need to breathe for (or "ventilate") the patient.

Anesthesia

Anesthesia is the loss of sensation which brings with it analgesia, loss of pain. In the absence of anesthesia other than a gulp of brandy or laudanum (an opium tincture popular at the time), which provided only incomplete and temporary relief, it was necessary to perform excruciating operative procedures in only a few minutes. Would you lie peacefully while someone cut open your chest? Before anesthesia, surgeons typically had to restrain the agonizing and thrashing patients with a combination of shackles and assistants.

Speed was a useful surgical attribute to minimize the challenge to the patient's fortitude. However, these hasty operations led to some unfortunate outcomes, such as the incident reported by Power and Liston of a mid-nineteenth century London surgeon, well known for his speed in leg amputation who "included both testes of his patient and two fingers of his assistant with a single swoop of the knife and flash of the saw." Even now, surgeons must be careful not to allow a preoccupation with speed to preempt precision and the gentleness to tissues, as emphasized by Mr. Belsey.

Physicians and surgeons in the eighteenth-century compressed tissues to alleviate pain during operations. This sends nerve signals to the brain which compete with pain messages, and does have some modest effectiveness: why else would we have the instinct to grab and squeeze an injured part of our body? But this does little to mitigate severe pain. Even hypnotism was tried, with anecdotal success. James Esdaile, a Scottish surgeon, claimed to have used hypnotism to perform 261 painless operations on Hindu patients in India. However, upon returning home he found, as described by Bishop, that "his hard-headed countrymen were far less impressionable."

Horrific stories of surgical patients' agony before anesthesia abound. Snow gives us a representative example of a Parisian lady who describes undergoing a mastectomy in her home without anesthetic support: "When the dreadful steel was plunged into the breast.... I needed no injunction not to restrain my cries. I began a scream that lasted ... during the whole time of the incision ... so excruciating was the agony.... I then felt the Knife ... against the breast bone—scraping it ...! When all was done ... I then saw Dr. Larry, pale nearly as myself, his face streaked with blood, & his expression depicting grief, apprehension, & almost horror." Surely this approached the limits of human endurance (patient) and tolerance for causing pain (surgeon).

Surgeons and patients needed true general anesthesia—and its two salutary effects. The first and most obvious benefit is that the patient is spared the torture of having to be awake and fully aware during a lengthy and invasive operation. The other is that the surgeon can take the time necessary to perform a precise and careful procedure. The patient is no longer a moving target, and not at risk of literally dying of the shock caused by the pain itself or brought about by blood loss the surgeon does not have time to staunch. A potential anesthetic, nitrous oxide, popularly known as laughing gas, was discovered in 1772 by the chemist Joseph Priestley. Another renowned chemist Humphrey Davy tried it on himself and found it relieved both a headache and a toothache. In 1800, Davy suggested its use in surgery, but his advice was not heeded. This was perhaps because he was a physicist and not a physician. The medical community may be forgiven for being unaware of Davy's formidably entitled treatise, *Researches, Chemical and Philosophical— Chiefly Concerning Nitrous Oxide or Dephlogisticated Air and its Respiration.* ("Dephlogisticated" refers to the belief at that time that a combustible, fire-like element called "phlogiston" was released when a substance burned.) Also, the choice of terminology was not felicitous; how seriously could one take a recommendation for something called "laughing gas"?

Not long after these events it was observed, probably by Davy's assistant Michael Faraday, that inhaling the vapor of liquid ether had anesthetic effects similar to nitrous oxide. For years, however, the only routine use of ether was getting high at parties. These activities were called "ether frolics," undermining our stereotype of staid and stodgy Victorian ladies and gentlemen; picture the human equivalent of bumper cars. In January 1842, the physician William Clarke regained his wits after frolicking only to find he had painlessly acquired bruises. Inspired by his experience, he went on successfully to use ether to anesthetize a patient while extracting a tooth. The frolicking craze became international as in March of the same year, Crawford Long, a physician in Georgia, and another frolic aficionado, used ether while painlessly excising a patient's neck tumor. Encouraged by the results, he proceeded to use it with other patients. These operations are well documented; however, because Long delayed publishing his experiences until 1848, he lost the race to claim priority despite actually being the first to employ ether in an operation.

In 1844, a dentist in Connecticut named Horace Wells attended a nitrous oxide demonstration and was impressed enough that he used it on himself when he had a colleague extract one of his teeth. He was so pleased with his pain-free experience that he conducted an exhibition at Massachusetts General Hospital, but the patient "groaned" during the dental extraction and the procedure was deemed a failure. Next up was Wells's pupil William Morton. Buoyed by his own experiences with ether, he convinced Massachusetts General's renowned chief of surgery John Collins Warren (a former student of Philip Physick) to give it another chance. Four years after Long's operation, Warren excised a neck tumor from a patient in October 1846 with Morton serving as the anesthetist. The patient lay quietly and without complaints during the operation; Warren famously declared ether anesthesia to be "no humbug." The medical community was made aware of this and several more successful pain-free operations by a November 1846 article in the *Boston Medical and Surgical Journal,* entitled "Insensibility During Surgical Operations Produced by Inhalation," which ushered in the era of general anesthesia. Morton notably went on to administer ether for battlefield operations during the Civil War, providing anesthesia during surgery for wounded Confederate soldiers. A disappointing final footnote is that Morton unsuccessfully spent the remainder of his life seeking to patent the anesthetic process, and thereby make his fortune.

Chloroform, an alternative inhalation agent, was introduced soon thereafter but its popularity was short-lived. It was more potent than ether but also more dangerous because it irritated the heart and caused lethal disruptions of its normal rhythm. It soon passed from favor. During its temporary popularity, however, it was used in the British Isles to alleviate the pain of childbirth. A resistance group raised the theological argument that mothers should suffer as part of Eve's punishment described in the Biblical injunction that "in sorrow thou shalt bring forth children." This was rebutted with the observation that the Lord caused a deep sleep to fall over Adam when harvesting the rib that was to become Eve. Opposition finally ceased when Queen Victoria used chloroform to ease her 1853 delivery.

As their specialty evolved from the ether and chloroform beginnings, anesthetists developed newer gas agents to induce a state of general anesthesia. They also have added a variety of potent intravenous drugs and added muscle relaxants so that the patient is not only asleep but also completely flaccid. This ensures that surgeons encounter no resistance to retraction of tissues; operations are safer as assistants can fully expose internal organs. Dissections of organs are enhanced by ease of access and unrestricted visibility. The modern anesthetist now has this extensive array of agents, so surgeons conduct operations on an unconscious, fully relaxed, and pain-free patient.

Surgeons had to have been energized by the evolving ability to induce general anesthesia. The anesthesia era enabled surgeons to operate inside the abdomen without the need to lash the patient down or proceed so hastily that mistakes were inevitable. Procedures in the chest, however, offered an unexpected challenge—breathing. What could be more automatic? Yet compensating for the patient's inability to perform this deceptively simple act was an unforeseen hurdle for thoracic surgery and the new profession of anesthesiology.

Ventilation

For a surgeon to get to the lungs and esophagus a thoracotomy is needed, the so-called "cracking" of the chest. This adds a challenge beyond general anesthesia goals of loss of sensation and pain: how can the patient breathe? The essential first steps were to figure out what the lungs did and how they did it. Early speculations were that the lung's role was to cool the blood to balance the heat introduced by the heart. Galen stood this on its head by asserting: "Blood passing through the lungs absorbed from the inhaled air, the quality of heat, which it then carried into the left heart."

There were more accurate insights by the fifteenth century. Leonardo wrote, "From the heart, impurities or sooty vapors are carried back to the lung by way of the pulmonary artery, to be exhaled to the outer air." William Harvey, famous for determining the role of the heart and the vascular system of arteries and veins, was on the right track when he observed, "Life and respiration are complementary. There is nothing living which does not breathe nor anything which breathing does not live." Eventually Priestley discovered oxygen, and the process of oxygen exchange for carbon dioxide was worked out.

So, oxygen and carbon dioxide are exchanged, but how does the air get in and out? It's not a passive process. When we breathe in, we use chest wall muscles to expand the chest. Simultaneously the diaphragm, also a muscle, contracts and descends to further enlarge the chest cavity—which is airless. This closed space is a vacuum; as it enlarges, it decreases the pressure inside it. The negative pressure expands the compliant lungs by drawing them outward. The negative pressure literally sucks oxygen-containing air into the lungs through the trachea or windpipe. When we breathe out, the process reverses. The chest wall and diaphragm muscles squeeze inward, closing the chest down, increasing pressure, compressing the lungs, and exhaling the air.

As emphasized in Chapter Four, this process won't work without an intact, inviolate chest cavity. A thoracotomy disrupts our normal breathing mechanism: the chest cavity is no longer a closed space, and negative pressure can no longer be generated. When the chest is open to the air, the vacuum and negative pleural pressure are lost; the lung's elastic tissues contract and collapse the lung. General anesthesia had arrived, but chest surgeons still needed a way to breathe for the patient with an open chest. There were two possible solutions. One was somehow to mimic normal physiology and generate negative pleural pressure to prevent lung collapse during a thoracotomy, allowing normal breathing to continue. The other was to find a way to *force* air into the lungs; a method called positive pressure ventilation.

Ferdinand Sauerbruch, an influential German surgeon, pursued the first option early in the twentieth century. He devised a negative pressure operating chamber which accommodated both the operating team and a patient whose head was outside the chamber. The patient breathed normally, and the negative pressure environment inside the chamber kept the patient's lungs expanded. This technique worked but was cumbersome, complicated, and expensive. It is more effective to ventilate the patient, forcing air under positive pressure into the trachea and lungs. Sauerbruch's technique of negative-pressure artificial ventilation was, however, eventually useful in later years with the so-called "iron lungs," which sustained paralyzed polio victims who were unable to breathe for themselves.

Vesalius, the previously mentioned anatomist, in 1543 had been the first to use positive pressure ventilation. Vesalius found that positive pressure ventilation was viable by keeping pigs alive during a thoracotomy by breathing for them through a reed inserted into a tracheotomy, a surgically created opening in the trachea in the neck. Other investigators duplicated this maneuver in animals, and in 1869 Trendelenburg used the technique with a human patient he ventilated through a tube inserted into a tracheotomy to prevent blood from draining into the lungs during an operation. William Macewen in 1880, in Scotland, was the first surgeon to *intubate* the trachea by passing a tube directly through the mouth. This intubation technique was an important innovation as it eliminated the need for a tracheotomy.

Surgeons began to catch on and started to utilize positive pressure ventilation, following Macewen's precedent, and intubating the trachea during surgery. A crude bellows powered by hand or foot pedals replaced the surgeon's lungs and was used to provide the positive pressure. Surgeons and anesthesiologists gained experience during World War I as they routinely used positive pressure endotracheal anesthesia during operations. Soon mechanical ventilators were developed to replace manual powering, freeing the anesthesiologist to focus all attention on the patient's care.

Increasingly sophisticated positive pressure ventilators are now ubiquitous in operating rooms and intensive care units. Thoracic surgeons can now safely open chests as patients are both anesthetized *and* effectively ventilated during a thoracotomy. With the essentials in place, two remaining surgical challenges could not be ignored: pain and infection.

7

PAIN AND
INFECTION

Pain

The operation ends, and the surgeon is content; the operation was performed in ideal conditions. The patient was asleep and fully relaxed. But it's not over for the patient—they are going to hurt. Analgesia is now the need. Surgical wards in hospitals are filled with patients craving pain relief as are those recovering at home as insurers demand early discharge from the hospital. I don't remember noticing this during my student days, but I certainly was well aware of it during my residency and practice years. Yet surprisingly, when walking surgical wards, I was not subjected to a chorus of moans; rather there was mainly the sounds of nurses at work, the beeping of various machines, and, in later years, the clacking of computer keyboards. After most operations—and certainly a thoracotomy—patients want to lie still and only take shallow breaths. It hurts to move, especially the chest. As I hope you would assume, surgeons care and worry about their suffering patients. But it's not just a humanitarian concern.

Become conscious of how often you take an occasional, involuntary deep breath, sigh, and even cough. All of these are activities retarded by chest pain. Without these actions, the lung's elastic tissue "squeeze" causes a tendency toward collapse. According to something called the Law of Laplace, it becomes progressively harder to re-expand as the lung shrinks down; easier to keep fully inflated or re-inflate small areas of collapse. Our involuntary actions pop back open small areas of collapse. The post-operative thoracotomy patient is at risk of progressive collapse because the pain of chest movement prevents deep breathing and coughing. Persistent or progressive consolidation can result in pneumonia and, in extreme circumstances, start the patient on a fatal spiral downward. Analgesia to diminish the chest pain helps the patient take deep breaths and cough enough to thwart this scenario.

I began all patients on a narcotic or narcotic-like drug after a thoracotomy. During my first years a nurse administered the drug intravenously. A helpful later innovation was a device the patient controlled to administer the drug; a scheme called PCA for "patient-controlled analgesia." The amount available over time was limited, and not each push of the switch contained the narcotic. The patients did not know when the drug was dispensed so they benefited from a placebo effect which supplemented the benefit of the narcotic. Titration of the amount was important as the goal was pain mitigation without actually putting the patient to sleep. Excess sedation is as detrimental as insufficient pain relief; the drowsy patient is equally unlikely to perform the deep breathing and coughing necessary to keep lungs fully inflated. To supplement the intravenous agents, before the operation the anesthesiologist usually inserted a catheter into the spinal canal through which narcotics could be instilled. These provided pain relief without affecting the patient's sensorium. There were drawbacks as this prevented the patient from feeling the need to urinate, so they needed a Foley catheter. The patient was monitored in the Intensive Care Unit as if the narcotic delivery was excessive it could suppress breathing.

I switched to an oral equivalent over the first few days which continued when the patient went home. Most patients were free of narcotics within a month. I allowed continuation up to six weeks but after that referred patients who expressed continuing pain to a pain management specialist. These specialists use many techniques for pain relief and are better able to distinguish real pain from a developing opioid addiction.

Thoracic surgeons have modified operative technique with the goal of preventing or at least mitigating postoperative pain. ("Cracking chests" didn't come out of nowhere). An important driver of pain after a thoracotomy is two ends of a broken rib rubbing against each other. The thoracic surgeon can break ribs when spreading them apart. This requires balancing that concern against the need to obtain adequate visualization of the operative field. I regularly removed a small segment of a rib; this was a deliberate fracture but kept the rib ends apart so they could not abrade each other. Some of my colleagues espoused another operative maneuver: retracting muscles of the chest wall out of the way to lessen pain rather than cutting through them. Both operative modifications seemed to be effective in some patients but neither consistently nor dramatically. The ultimate surgical modification seems to have arrived in the form of minimally invasive operations.

An open surgical procedure in the abdomen is a laparotomy— a misnomer for an abdominal incision as it is derived from the Greek "lapara" for flank. In the chest, it's a thoracotomy. During these operations, the incision is spread open and held apart by metal retractors. The advent of minimally invasive surgery didn't just shift this historic paradigm; it created an entirely new one. I admit I never saw this remarkable innovation in surgical technique coming. A minimally invasive operation is identified by appending the suffix "-*oscopy*" to the name of the appropriate body part; for the chest a thoracoscopy, for the abdomen a laparoscopy. Only a few short cuts in the skin of about one centimeter (about one-third of an inch) are necessary. The surgeon inserts tubular devices called "ports" through the incisions and through them passes a video camera and operating instruments which are much longer than standard instruments. During a thoracoscopic procedure the anesthesiologist uses a special breathing tube which allows ventilation of only the lung on the opposite side from the operation. This allows the lung on the operated side to collapse. The ribs support the chest wall so as the lung falls away space is created for the surgeon to maneuver instruments. The abdomen, in contrast, lacks this supporting bony structure. To provide room to wield surgical tools during a laparoscopic operation, carbon dioxide gas is instilled through a port with enough pressure to distend the abdominal cavity.

Although there was initial controversy regarding the safety and efficaciousness of replacing the gold standard of traditional open surgery with this quite different methodology, minimally invasive approaches are now commonly used and have taken their place as the standard technique for many major operations. There are several benefits from the patient's perspective which contribute to its popularity compared to the traditional open-operative technique. As its name implies, the patient has much less pain after a less invasive operation as the trauma to skin and muscle of a few short incisions is less than that associated with a single but much longer cut. The cosmetic results are superior as the relatively lengthy and typically visible scar following an open operation is replaced with a few short ones that tend to disappear in skin folds and be hidden under hair.

Finally, an unexpected boon for both patient and surgeon is that minimally invasive procedures stimulate the inflammatory system much less than open ones, reducing patient stress by several orders of magnitude. This translates into a reduction of peri-operative morbidity, quicker recovery, and the ability for the patient to return sooner to work (perhaps a mixed blessing) and normal life activities. In the field of thoracic surgery, thoracoscopic techniques for both lung and esophageal operations have only relatively recently been established as safe and effective in curing cancer. When minimally invasive operations were first performed, surgeons worried that blood loss from a significant injury to an artery might actually prove fatal to a patient. The feared scenario was an excessive delay in finding and closing the arterial defect as accumulated blood obscured camera visibility so that a hastily performed emergency thoracotomy or laparotomy was necessary; it takes some time to cut through skin and muscle and spread the ribs apart, perhaps enough time for a patient to exsanguinate. However, the development of thoracoscopic surgery has been led by careful and conservative surgeons who have matured the techniques so that minimally invasive operations in the hands of experienced surgeons are as safe as open operations and bring the benefits previously identified.

Infection

Anesthesia, including the ability to ventilate an unconscious patient, made thoracic surgery possible. Analgesic drugs made it tolerable. But the surgical ship sailed with unrecognized stowaways: bacteria. They were the unknown and, indeed, unimagined challengers to reliably good outcomes. Infection became the *bête noire* of invasive operations. It's frustrating for surgeons and harmful for patients to complete a seemingly successful operation only to have an infection develop in the wound or inside the abdomen or chest; this complicates recovery and can be life-threatening.

But you can't fight the enemy until it's identified. Many recall the story of the Dutchman Antonie van Leeuwenhoek who, in the late seventeenth century, used powerful microscopes he designed and manufactured to catch sight of one-celled microorganisms he called *animalcules,* which just means "little organisms." His finding of what we now know as bacteria or germs made it possible to refute science's longstanding belief in spontaneous generation, a notion attributed to Aristotle that organisms could arise spontaneously from putrid meat or even a pile of dirty rags.

Leeuwenhoek spotted the animalcules, but what did they do? Several scientists, most famously Louis Pasteur in the mid-nineteenth century, began to answer. He found that boiled broths exposed to the air became cloudy, proof of infestation by something unseen, whereas identical preparations excluded from the air and airborne microorganisms, such as those identified by Leeuwenhoek, remained clear. The enemy had been found, identifying the target for methods of antisepsis.

At roughly the same time as Louis Pasteur proved microorganisms rather than "miasma" or spontaneous generation were responsible for infection, Ignaz Semmelweis, a physician in Vienna, provided not only further evidence supporting the germ theory, but a lifesaving surgical improvement for pregnant women: he required physicians under his supervision to *wash their hands* prior to delivering babies. He instituted this "radical" demand after observing that pregnant women delivered by physicians who had just autopsied an infected person had a much higher rate of uterine infection (puerperal sepsis) than pregnant women delivered by midwives with uncontaminated hands. The result was a dramatic reduction in new mothers' puerperal infection rate which fell from 18% to 2.2% in Semmelweis' hospital. Yet his empirically better practice was rejected by the Viennese medical establishment because it ran counter to their locked-in belief that "miasma" or bad air caused infections. Physicians also resisted handwashing as gentlemen whose social standing alone, they believed, was sufficient to ensure cleanliness. (Puerperal sepsis was a frequent complication of childbirth. It is thought to have killed Jane Seymour, Henry VIII's third wife. Several heads might have remained in place if her physician had only washed his hands.). Semmelweis was so devastated by his colleagues' obstinacy that he ended up in an insane asylum. His death shortly after admission was, ironically, probably due to a gangrenous infection contracted after asylum guards administered a beating.

European physicians and surgeons finally began to recognize the truth (and implications) of the germ theory when Joseph Lister, a surgeon in Glasgow in the 1860s, called for the use of a carbolic acid spray (a bactericidal phenol solution) on all surgical instruments and the patient's skin. He showed that saturating wound dressings with a carbolic acid solution greatly reduced the rate of wound infection following treatment of compound fractures, which are those with bone fragments protruding through the skin. Lister, who also advocated washing instruments and the wearing of clean clothes by surgeons, derived his idea for the use of carbolic acid from the observation that the polluted Clyde River in Glasgow appeared clear where phenol from a nearby chemical plant drained into it. The germ theory was becoming germ science.

One of his successes was to use this solution to save the poet William Ernest Henley's leg from amputation. Henley had a tubercular infection of his shin bone, or tibia, and endured a 21-month hospitalization which included frequent wound debridements which required daily scraping of his bone and changes of his carbolic acid-soaked wound dressing. We may imagine that suffering yet surviving this excruciating experience inspired Henley's famous poem, "Invictus," a paean to defiant self-reliance in the face of the "fell clutch of circumstance."

American surgeons were initially unimpressed by Pasteur's and Lister's evidence and results from across the sea. Their resistance is illustrated by the famous 1875 painting of the Gross Clinic which depicts Dr. Gross, a leading light in the Philadelphia surgical community, operating surrounded by students to whom he is lecturing, and assistants who are restraining the patient. No antiseptic techniques are in evidence. Dr. Gross's hands and his scalpel are blood-stained; he wears neither gloves nor mask and is in his street clothes. There is no evidence of an antibacterial solution on the patient. The patient is at risk of infection from bacteria on the surgeon, the instruments and even his own skin. Happily, Lister's speeches about and demonstrations of his principles during a tour of America in 1876 are credited with turning the surgical tide in favor of their acceptance by skeptical American surgeons.

Currently, operating room personnel are well attuned to the need for antisepsis in their environment. Carbolic acid has been superseded by autoclaving instruments, which sterilizes them with heat. Surgeons wear clean "scrubs" rather than blood-stained three-piece suits; cleaning and sterilization of the patients' skin are routine components of any surgical procedure. We surgeons also wear masks to block transmission of pharyngeal bacteria, and surgical gloves serve as a barrier between our patients and the bacteria on our skin and under our fingernails. Even the most vigorous scrubbing can never make skin sterile although it does reduce the bacterial population. Surprisingly, gloves were not originally intended for this purpose. They were famously introduced by William Halsted to protect the hands of his scrub nurse and future wife from the irritating carbolic acid. There is room for love in surgery.

Operating rooms are now zealously scrubbed between operations, and bactericidal agents are sprayed on wall, floors, and all furniture. Finally, antibiotics, starting with the sulfonamides in the 1930s (put to good use in World War II), and penicillin in 1944, are now in common use. The obvious reason is to treat active infections. This has greatly benefited patients with infections such as pneumonia. Equally important is their prophylactic use in patients undergoing operations to prevent development of infections afterward. Bacteria are everywhere. We paint the patient's skin with bactericidal solutions, wash our hands and wear masks; actions designed to diminish bacteria's numbers on skin and protect from the surgeon's mouth and nose. But some linger on; you can't sterilize skin. Tissues in the wound are exposed to these bacteria. In addition, the patient's own internal organs such as the gastrointestinal tract are teeming with bacteria. For chest surgeries, the concern is when a surgeon cuts into the lungs or esophagus which also harbor bacteria. From all these sources, bacteria can infest and infect a wound and tissues exposed during surgery. Better to never have an infection than need to treat one; the appropriate use of prophylactic antibiotics to eradicate these potential contaminants has prevented many an infection.

It is important, however, to be judicious in the use of antibiotics; there can be too much of a good thing. Bacteria resistant to the antibiotics emerge if their use is prolonged. The ideal is to give them intravenously as the operation begins and stop within a few hours after the procedure ends. There is another unintended consequence of lengthy usage. The drugs go everywhere in the body; they are not limited to the operative site. The antibiotics begin to wipe out the normal bacteria in the intestines, what is called the human microbiome. This altered microbiome can result in diarrhea ranging in severity from mild to bloody and life-threatening.

Washing your hands; simple but effective. As Semmelweis observed, reducing the bacterial load on your hands by doing what your mother insisted on has a major impact on the development of infections. Although handwashing by surgeons prior to donning sterile gloves has been standard for the last century, only in the last few *decades* has it become hospital policy in America to require physicians and nurses to wash and decontaminate their hands between patient encounters on the hospital floors. This practice has long been recommended but only recently has the policy been strongly enforced.

I wish I could claim my patients never developed an infection after an operation. Not so. There has been a change in where infecting bacteria come from after chest operations. With all the attention paid to surgeon attire and handwashing, sterilizing the patient's skin, and prophylactic antibiotics, an infection now frequently means an esophageal anastomosis is leaking. I'll talk more about this when I discuss esophageal cancer.

8

▼

FACULTY

As I neared the end of my residency in thoracic surgery, I continued to feel certain I wanted to remain in academia rather than go into private practice. Accordingly, I began to interview with medical schools for a faculty position in thoracic surgery. I was a reasonably competitive candidate: I had presented my research findings at national surgical societies, published in surgical journals, and had my bona fides from my training at the University of Chicago. At this point, most hospitals and medical schools still combined cardiac and general thoracic chest surgeons into a cardiothoracic group with an emphasis on heart procedures. Not surprising; coronary artery bypass operations were being performed by the thousands, the demand was incessant, and the economic rewards were considerable.

I was looking for a faculty position at the time these groups were realizing their general thoracic expertise was lagging behind the cardiac. I returned perplexed from my interviews with several academic departments of surgery—all positions had attractive aspects, but none was ideal. Some required more participation in cardiac surgery than interested me. A few wanted to task me with developing their thoracic program but without the support of similarly inclined colleagues. Indecision was put to rest when Dr. Skinner summoned me to his office and offered me a position as an assistant professor in his department. Perfect. I accepted eagerly, pleased to be able to stay home but with the fleeting concern of developing my own practice as I found myself in competition for patients with the aforementioned greats.

What attracted about academia? Why not private practice? Perhaps wanting to be an academic surgeon seems pretentious. Not meant to be. It simply means being on the faculty of a medical school and its department of surgery. Academic surgeons are actively practicing surgeons but also are teachers and researchers. This variety of activities appealed to me. Some surgeons in private practice have a relationship with a medical school and participate in teaching and training medical students and surgical residents, but most are fully occupied with their clinical practice. I liked the wide spectrum of academic activities that came with being on the faculty of a medical school and its department of surgery. The opportunity to be part of a university culture also appealed.

Academic surgeons of all specialties do routine procedures but are also frequently sought to provide care for patients with advanced cancers (those invading adjacent tissues or involving lymph nodes) or complications from previous operations. Advanced cancers require extensive resections, including surrounding tissue and lymph nodes, to get all the cancer. The surgeon is challenged by reoperations because of adhesions (internal scarring binding organs together and obscuring normal anatomic tissue planes), which are the residual effects of dissections during earlier operations (what Belsey called "muddy footprints"). These are complex surgical interventions which academic surgeons seek out—because we like the challenge, not because of masochism. Medical school surgeons also pursue their scholarly interests, teach medical students, and train surgery residents. They are on the cutting edge (an unavoidable pun) as they work to advance the capabilities of the specialty. Our goal is to translate our experiences and investigations into insights that mature into new treatment algorithms or alternative surgical techniques to improve patient outcomes.

I should mention a "town-gown" scenario that sometimes arises—a family quarrel. It usually takes the form of a mild and trivial rivalry between academic and private-practice medical communities, but occasionally breaks out into highly competitive disputes over perceptions of who works the hardest, or real-world concerns such as control of a hospital staff. This observation will be relevant in the chapter about my Las Vegas experience.

A common misconception of patients is the belief that physicians in academic medical centers are drooling at the chance to experiment on them. Therefore, they avoid university hospitals with might and main. I admit that as recently as when I was a resident, I knew of patients who were entered into clinical trials without their knowledge or consent. These were well-intended investigations by physicians who wanted to answer an important clinical question without putting the patient at risk. Nonetheless, it was inappropriate, as the patients were unaware. Those days are long over. Oversight committees called Institutional Review Boards (IRB) are now required in all hospitals where clinical studies are performed. All investigations into any aspect of patient care—such as comparing a new drug to an old one, or an innovative new operation to improve on the current standard—are thoroughly vetted by the IRB both to ensure they are safe for patients, to be sure the clinical question being asked is actually scientifically valid, and that the study is designed so as to bring home an answer. Of course, all patients who are prospective study subjects must have the rationale for, and details of, the study, as well as the implications of their participation, including all risks, explained to them. They sign a consent form documenting these steps were followed and reminding them they can withdraw from the study at any time. The IRB constantly monitors the study to ensure continued patient safety. No one gets surreptitiously experimented on.

I didn't really have a clue about "academia," being a faculty member of a university, while I was a medical student. My father was in private practice and that was all I knew. During residency I became aware the faculty surgeons at Hopkins and Chicago were researchers as well as clinicians, some in laboratories and others analyzing patient experiences, in addition to their routine of operations and daily care of patients. My curiosity grew and led to my research year at Chicago. That experience captured me; I wanted to help the specialty develop. I also realized there were other aspects of academia, in addition to research and taking care of patients, which had a great deal of appeal: teaching and training medical students and residents; transforming them from raw neophytes into the mature physicians who form the workforce of the future. Performing a successful operation on one patient is an important contribution but to the health of only one person. Improving operations, adding new understanding of disease processes, or developing new procedures or ways to enhance patient care, when adopted by other surgeons, multiplies the contribution going forward to many patients.

Therefore, participating in national societies where the results of basic or clinical research studies are presented to a large audience of surgeons or publishing them in surgical journals is critical. This is how information is disseminated. The surgeons attending the conferences or reading the journals consider the study, particularly the validity of its methods and the credibility of its results and evaluate the new data from the perspective of their own experience with the same type of patients as those in the study. Depending on the outcome of this process, the recommendations of the study (perhaps a new operation or one operation where several alternatives exist) are put into practice or used to identify operations or patterns of patient care that should be abandoned. The clinical world is constantly changing and the information from these studies provides the scaffolding on which the new is built.

A challenge for medical school faculty when it comes to medical students is to develop empathy—to consider students' long-term goals. If you are a surgeon, it's important to realize that most of your students are aiming toward a career in another discipline. Less than 10 percent of students end in a surgical specialty. It is a bad idea to try to use the few weeks of the experience of the third year of medical school to lure a student into a surgical career; this can be tempting when the talents of a superior student catch your eye. However, if the choice of specialty is not made organically, the student may ultimately find themselves discontented either during their residency, incentivizing them to switch residencies, or even later in their practice when it is too late to change fields. This is good for neither the student nor the specialty. Faculty must make sure students have a sufficient exposure to all disciplines so that they can make an informed decision as to their eventual careers. When a student is interested in surgery, they will go through a surgical residency for education and training. My goal for the medical student choosing a non-surgical career was to provide an understanding of diseases that require surgical intervention. I wanted them to know how best to evaluate and manage a patient while obtaining the participation of a surgeon, and how to identify patients who need urgent surgical care. On the positive side, all are motivated and eager to learn, a characterization I suspect many teachers of younger students would envy.

I was never disappointed in my decision to remain at the University of Chicago. One reason was the opportunity to participate in the multi-specialty group that DeMeester had organized with the Chief of Medical Oncology to coordinate the care of patients with cancers of the chest. The Chest Oncology Group was ahead of its time; a model program, academia at its best. A consortium of thoracic surgeons, medical oncologists, radiologists, and pulmonologists met weekly to review, discuss, debate, and, ultimately, determine the treatment plan for patients with lung or esophageal cancer. This multi-disciplinary process obviated the all-too-common scenario of a patient receiving treatment provided by the specialist they first happened to see. (The relevant joke is that if you go to a barber, you are likely to get a haircut.) It also meant that patient care decisions were informed by the input of multiple opinions and full consideration of alternative therapeutic options.

This arrangement also provided the platform for us to carry out studies to evaluate new patient care strategies. When there is uncertainty about a particular care strategy for a disease, for example, when a new strategy seems to offer an improvement, answers are sought by comparing the alternative approaches. This is essential in determining the role and efficacy of a new treatment, be it a drug or operation, and is a prime example of the benefit of activities within academia. Under the watchful eye of the IRB, our multi-specialty group set up studies comparing the current standard therapies to new options, then analyzed the results of the trials. We randomly distributed patients into the two groups being treated with one of the two therapies, so that the two groups' members were similar and comparing them was valid. For example, we studied the potential benefit of giving the patient chemotherapy or radiation therapy before operating for esophageal cancer. Administering a therapy prior to an operation is called "neoadjuvant therapy," because adjuvant therapy is administered after an operation; it was not standard. Half the patients got the neoadjuvant therapy, and half did not. It turned out this strategy does improve the ability to cure the patient in most circumstances, but there were complications associated with combining all these therapies. This is a conundrum still being evaluated in many academic centers—risks versus benefits.

Learning to organize and lead these types of studies as part of the University of Chicago's Chest Oncology Group was a valuable part of my development as an academic surgeon. The benefit for me was not just academic. As a result of my participation in the Group, I was able to operate on a regular basis on patients with lung or esophageal cancer. Resections for these two cancers are now a routine thoracic surgical undertaking; however, this was not always the case. In later chapters, we'll explore the steps in the development of lung and esophageal surgery and the surgeons who led the way.

So, for me academia was a flame, and I was a moth. But I was a surgeon; caring for patients—which, for a surgeon, means operating on them—was my primary interest. As the junior faculty member in the Thoracic Surgery Division in Chicago, I had no administrative responsibilities. Teaching and mentoring took little "extra" time as they were integrated into the normal clinical activities of operating and making rounds to check on patients. This left me free to devote myself to two principal activities. The first was to develop my clinical practice and solidify my confidence that I was capable of independently caring for patients who required major thoracic operations. For that I needed patients; the challenge was to convince my colleagues in medicine to refer patients to me. I followed the recommended strategy of adhering to the three As, in this order: availability, affability, and ability. Patients rarely come directly to a surgeon; they are referred by a physician from a different specialty, for example, an oncologist. So, if a physician attempts a referral and the surgeon does not respond, the physician's calls will quickly dry up (availability). Similarly, if the encounter with the surgeon is not pleasant, the same outcome can be expected (the second "a"). Finally, if patients do not do well after an operation, of course the referring physician will take that into account. I did my best to stick to these precepts and as time went along, I experienced growth in my practice; patients began to appear.

Stories of representative patients on whom I operated for cancer I'll share in the chapters on lung and esophageal cancer. I'm occasionally asked if being a surgeon for patients with these grim cancers wasn't depressing. It wasn't because I had a chance to cure them. Patients with metastatic disease or who are too frail for an operation are cared for by medical oncologists. My operations did not always result in a long-term cure, but it was always a possibility. Removal of an esophagus or lung is not done for short-term palliation. Only if there is a realistic chance of cure should a surgeon put a patient through the challenges of tolerating a major operation.

Not all operations are for cancer. I frequently operated, for example, for GERD, simply to improve the quality of someone's life. Perhaps performing surgery to make someone feel better sounds frivolous, but not to a person with heartburn that is intensely painful, wakes them at night, restricts their diet—no coffee, tea, chocolate, or alcohol—and requires them to sleep with the head of their bed elevated. Depending on several factors, including the patient's size and how badly the acid reflux had damaged the esophagus, I operated through either the chest or abdomen. These antireflux operations were gratifying; they were safe, effective, and resulted in happy patients. When they fail, I believe this is more due to operating on patients who don't actually have GERD than surgical skill and emphasizes the benefit of pH monitoring of the esophagus to confirm the reflux diagnosis.

During surgery, I was accompanied by a resident whom I was responsible for training. These were men and women—yep, women were beginning to take their rightful place in the specialty—who had completed five years of general surgery training. Technically, they were accomplished; they possessed the basic skills. For them, it was a matter of learning new operations. But that revealed a normal human characteristic: resistance to change. In a sense, humans tend to be conservative. Residents balked at using techniques that differed from what they had been taught as students or earlier in their residencies. Eventually most, like me, realized there were reasonable alternative methods and techniques, and becoming fluent with as many as possible only puts more arrows in your quiver.

I was now in the position of my surgical mentors: when I began to work with a resident, I performed most of the operations and supervised them as they incrementally assumed the primary surgeon role. This was a little frustrating, as I personally loved to operate but the reward was sharing the residents' growth of confidence as their skills improved. Things went well until my first serious complication. While performing a lung lobectomy (removal of part of the lung) for lung cancer, I demonstrated for the resident the technique for removing a group of lymph nodes from the mediastinum (the area between the lungs and behind the heart), a procedure I had performed dozens of times. Suddenly we found ourselves looking inside the esophagus. Not good. Unbeknownst to us the patient had a diverticulum, an outpouching, from the esophagus attached to the lymph nodes and I had cut across it. I was able to suture closed the hole in the esophagus which must have healed as the patient recovered uneventfully. But I worried for a week until he was out of danger. I learned two lessons from this experience, and others, as time passed. The first is that stuff happens. I do not mean to be cavalier, but, if you go around cutting on people there will be times when operations fail, infections develop, and even when patients die. Secondly, these outcomes are by no means always the surgeon's fault; but they always hurt as you feel responsible.

As a resident, I had been encouraged to "take ownership" of the patients we cared for—that is, to feel personally connected to and responsible for them. However, because we were residents, even though we operated on them, provided postoperative care, and entered into necessarily intense relationships with them and their families, they were not truly *our* patients or responsibility.

As happens to all surgeons after residency I realized that now, my patients were truly *mine*. I met them in the office to discuss their disease and the risks and benefits of a surgical procedure, operated on them, and supervised their postoperative recovery. This intensely personal connection amplified the empathy and sense of responsibility well beyond what I had already felt as a resident. I don't think a patient would or should expect anything less than having their surgeon feel personally and totally bonded to them.

Clinical activity, seeing patients in my office and operating on them, was a consistent activity. Teaching and training medical students and residents was, and would remain, a constant thread in the fabric of my life as an academic surgeon. Now, I came face to face with the fact that no one had taught me to be a teacher or mentor. As I became responsible for teaching students in their third year I realized I didn't know basic educational principles. I had been a student but converting to the teacher role was a challenge. I lectured to students only enough to realize that was not the best educational technique. During my student experience, I had not realized how inefficient lectures were. Watching my sleep-deprived students drift off as I spoke to them led me to adopt what is called a problem-based learning technique. Students are given a patient scenario and then the group dissects and analyzes questions of diagnosis and treatment. They must think and actually use the facts the previous two years packed into them; all are alert and engaged. And more is learned and retained than by a soporific lecture.

It was different with residents; classroom lectures were rare. We interacted in clinical settings. I came to understand that training young men and women to become mature and independent surgeons is mainly an art. The decision of when and how to permit a resident to assume the lead role in an operation is typically based on the teaching surgeon's personal assessment of and confidence in the technical skills, maturity, and judgment of any particular resident. When I was a resident, particularly a chief resident, I always wanted more opportunities in the operating room and was frustrated when it didn't come. Looking back and considering my internal struggles with deciding how much leeway to give residents under my wing I realize how judicious my teachers were. Despite their eagerness, I found most residents needed a slower and steadier progression through the operating process than they appreciated.

Early on, like my colleagues, I taught medical students using methods I picked up from my teachers and followed my instincts. Happily, educational research in recent years has brought us new insights that are informing the teaching and learning process by introducing scientific principles and making the process less subjective. It's a challenge to decide how much responsibility or even independence to allow residents in the throes of development of their skills and surgical judgment, especially in the operating room. It is true that due to the current mandates of several overseeing agencies, the attending surgeon must now always be present in the operating room and residents do not operate alone any longer. This requirement is patently reasonable—in fact, is overdue—as the attending surgeon is responsible for the patient's outcome. However, there is a delicate balance the teaching surgeon—as the most experienced surgeon in the operating room—must strike between doing all of an operation "from skin to skin" and allowing a resident to actively participate so they can develop their own independent capability.

Residents must assist and observe an experienced surgeon to develop their technical skills and an understanding of the operative algorithm for specific procedures; however, the residents must themselves perform a sufficient number of operations to become independent, safe, and self-reliant surgeons by the time their training ends and they begin their independent practice. Under current standards for supervision and teaching the resident serves as the operating surgeon under careful observation and guidance by the attending surgeon. The resident thus develops technique and confidence and participates actively, in a graduated fashion, as their ability progresses until they can demonstrate full mastery of a given procedure.

Education, however, is not all academia is about; in addition to teaching and mentoring, I needed to have a presence in the world of academic thoracic surgery. This meant sharing evidence of academic contributions in the form of articles for publication and talks at national surgical society meetings. The long-standing injunction to "publish or perish" is still relevant for those wishing to advance in any academic culture. It's frequently derided yet published articles and national presentations remain the measures of scholarly achievement.

The workings of surgical societies are similar to those of other academic disciplines. Surgeons submit brief abstracts containing the salient points of research or clinical experience to the surgical society for possible presentation at its annual meeting. A committee reviews these submissions and selects some for its annual meeting program.

Broadly speaking, there are two types of research studies. One analyzes the experience of a single surgeon or, more typically, a surgical group, with a particular disease or operation. This type of study may simply be a report of an experience accumulated over time: what was done and to whom, what were the results, and the authors' observations and conclusions.

In contrast to these clinical studies, the other type is more truly scientific. These may contain results of basic science laboratory experimentation or report results based on investigations in patients such as our efforts in Chicago to determine the esophageal function and acid reflux profiles of patients with GERD or motility disturbances. Both of these types of investigatory studies provide basic information that ideally can be "translated" into the clinical realm and affect patient care. At minimum, they yield useful biological information about diseases or normal functions that can inform clinical considerations.

If accepted by the committee, the surgeon presents the material in the study to attendees of the annual meeting. The speaker must compress the presentation of their research into a ten-minute talk, once upon a time with slides, now with a PowerPoint presentation. Surgical society meetings are well attended; discussion following each presentation ensures airing of multiple viewpoints, supportive and critical. Discussions are typically collegial and insightful; occasionally they become heated, as differences of opinion or interpretation arise. Occasionally arguments between presenter and discussant, both scientific and *ad hominem,* ensue. The presentation is fleshed out into a scientific article, providing more detail than was possible to cram into 10 minutes, and published in a surgical journal after further peer review. The discussions are published along with the eventual article, so readers are made aware of dissenting or critical commentary.

What is peer review? Review of one's research by a panel of one's surgical peers identifies information that is innovative (with the potential to influence surgical understanding of a disease or operation), and winnows out inaccurate, incomplete, or unimportant studies. The conclusions and recommendations of these studies could even be harmful, as professional publications can strongly influence other surgeons' selection of patients for a particular operation, and the technique chosen for a given procedure. This is also why Belsey emphasized keeping track of patients to be sure early results held up over time.

I found participating in the academic and social activities of society meetings, and being an active member of the society's committees, establishes a network of friends and colleagues. Participation was far from all business. Groups formed and met for dinner and the occasional beer. Friends would bring their friends and colleagues and relationships developed. Personal friendships blossomed; experiences were shared. This interaction was one of the pleasures of life in academia. For me, and all academic physicians, presenting at these conferences and publishing articles in the surgical journals was essential for promotion and career advancement. That always seemed appropriate to me: garnering the acceptance and respect of one's peers seemed a clear indication of being on the right track.

One final thought about academia; I've presented its workings as a smooth process: studies or experiences are presented and published, the community considers, and the wheel of progress turns. Let me nuance this a bit: clinical studies are subject to interpretation. Authors see their findings through the lenses of their biases and expectations. To my knowledge actual deliberate fraud is rare. But, for the above reasons, conclusions need to be put through the academic grinder: surgeons accrue other experiences, time goes by, and the truth ultimately emerges much less smoothly and much more slowly than the initial impression I may have given you.

9

SURGERY FOR GASTROESOPHAGEAL REFLUX DISEASE

Ambroise Paré, despite being the leading light of French surgery in the sixteenth century, was mystified. He was performing an autopsy of a man killed by a stabbing, when he "opened the belly [abdomen] and could not find the stomach [which] made … [him] … marvel greatly, thinking it a monstrous thing to be without a stomach." He continued to explore the abdomen and found that the wounding weapon had penetrated the diaphragm. He "realized that [the stomach] must have entered the thorax even though the wound in the diaphragm was no larger than enough to admit the thumb. On opening the thorax … [he] … found the stomach filled with air." Mystery solved; the stomach had simply herniated through the traumatic defect in the diaphragm into the chest.

I tell this story to emphasize that we can't figure out how or why a body part is malfunctioning unless we first understand its normal function. Paré was astounded, and *actually briefly able to imagine a person could live without a stomach.* Typical for the times, the necessity for and function of internal organs was frequently either unknown or misunderstood. The story of so-called "benign" esoph-ageal disease begins with exploring the anatomy and physiology of the normal, healthy esophagus.

The word "esophagus"—spelled oesophagus in Great Britain—is taken from the Greek *oisophagos* which combines *oisein* to carry, with *phagein* to eat. It was once commonly referred to as the gullet, as it still is in birds, from the Latin *gula* for throat. The esophagus actually contributes nothing to the digestive process. As detailed in Appendix Three, it is simply a biologic conveyer belt connecting mouth and stomach. Food is neither broken down into smaller bits nor absorbed during this transit. But it allows us to swallow food and get it where it can be digested. The esophagus is an active transport mechanism. Peristalsis, a sequence of contractions of the muscles of the esophagus, propels food from mouth to stomach, although gravity can speed up the transit of liquids. Swallowing is disrupted when this mechanism goes awry, causing the patient to have dysphagia, difficulty swallowing. Other important functional features of our esophagus are its two muscular sphincters that squeeze at the top where the esophagus departs from the pharynx, and at the bottom, where the esophagus joins the stomach. The top sphincter guards the pharynx and lungs by resisting regurgi-tation of esophageal contents. (The pharynx is at the back of the throat; it's the area from which the esophagus and the trachea arise. Regurgitated food can overflow into the trachea, where we can breathe it into our lungs. This is called "aspiration," and can cause pneumonia.) The lower sphincter serves as a barrier to protect the esophagus from acid reflux from the stomach. (For more anatomic and functional detail, see Appendix Three.)

The inconsistent terminology to describe the union of the esophagus and the stomach can be confusing to a patient. The most precise description is simply the gastroesophageal junction, also frequently referred to as the cardia (because this region is just behind the heart, *kardia* in Greek) which designates the terminal few centimeters of the esophagus as it joins the stomach. Finally, from a physiologic perspective the term lower esophageal sphincter is used to denote a high-pressure zone, the result of a muscular squeeze which can be detected at this location by esophageal manometry.

Gastroesophageal Reflux Disease (GERD)

The story of the development of surgical procedures for GERD is worth recounting in detail for several reasons. First, GERD is an extremely common cause of distress. Defining GERD is a little tricky as its predominant symptom (heartburn), caused by stomach acid heading upstream and irritating the esophagus, is quite common. But people with occasional heartburn don't have a disease. My definition of GERD is acid reflux which is bothersome enough for someone to consult a physician. Some 65 million prescriptions are written yearly for GERD and five percent of primary care visits are for this disease. It is estimated that 60% of adults have some GERD symptoms, principally heartburn and regurgitation of gastric contents into the mouth. These symptoms occur weekly in a third of these individuals.

The other reason to look into the development of surgical treatment of GERD is that the sequence of events—a tale with false starts and serendipity—is paradigmatic of the stepwise process by which the challenges of *disorders of function,* in contrast to *defects of anatomy,* are typically solved. This is an important distinction. In the case of GERD, the anatomy of the esophagus and stomach is normal; the organs have their normal relationship and there are no tumors. But things are not working as they should; the two organs are not functioning properly. Anatomic defects—think broken bones or a cancer—may challenge the surgeon to correct but are easy to spot. Functional disorders leave no such obvious footprints; identification requires putting together pieces of the puzzle such as symptoms and the results of tests of function such as manometry—is the esophageal muscle functioning properly?—and pH monitoring—is there an abnormal amount of acid reflux?

The first step for the surgeon is to be clear about what is "normal" or physiologic. When organs are functioning normally, life is good, and people feel well. Symptoms, feelings that all is not well, tell us some process has gone awry. We build on accumulated clinical experience with symptom-free people and symptomatic patients, supplemented by techniques for analysis, to determine pathophysiology (the way in which normal becomes deranged): What and how is the malfunction?

We clinicians inevitably make missteps and there are errors of interpretation along the way. As experience adds building blocks of understanding, we use them to evolve current operations or originate new ones for improved surgical results. Surgeons consider revising or adding operative techniques and make use of newer instruments. Over time, we develop increasingly satisfactory surgical options, resulting in more reliable and longer-lasting relief of symptoms. This is why it is important to have academic surgeons and their medical colleagues to innovate and then vet the innovations.

As regards GERD, thoracic surgery's initial misstep was focusing on the anatomy of hiatal hernia before we correctly identified acid reflux as a functional issue. A hernia is an abnormal protrusion of an internal organ through a defect in a muscle or into an anatomic opening. The most well-known is the groin hernia in which the small intestine herniates through a weak spot in the muscles of the abdominal wall. Surgeons have been repairing groin hernias for many years, in part because they hurt and are unsightly as they enlarge. However, the main driving force for correction is to prevent the development of two related complications: incarceration and strangulation. The former is a condition in which the herniating organ twists on itself or is squeezed by swollen tissues and becomes stuck (incarcerated) within the sac of *peritoneum*, the membrane lining the abdominal cavity. Incarceration progresses to strangulation when the intestine is not only stuck and unable to fall from the sac back into the abdomen, but its arterial blood supply is kinked or compressed so that there is insufficient flow to keep the herniated bowel segment alive. Necrosis or death of the herniated intestine is inevitable. Incarceration is a sign that strangulation is impending, and strangulation is a life-threatening condition. Without prompt surgical intervention to repair the hernia and return its contents to the abdomen or excise the bowel if it is necrotic and restore intestinal continuity, resulting infection will prove lethal as the intestine falls apart and releases its contents.

A hiatal hernia is a protrusion of the stomach upward and through the tissue membrane guarding the esophageal hiatus (the opening in the diaphragm through which the esophagus, descending from the throat, departs the chest to reach the stomach).

Some hiatal hernias are quite large and termed paraesophageal (because they are alongside the esophagus) or giant (because most or even all of the stomach is herniating), but these are fairly rare and not the ones that concern us here. The smaller and more common hernias are described as "sliding"—because the stomach slides up a short distance through the esophageal hiatus. These hernias are most likely the result of years of straining during bowel movements. This raises pressure within the abdomen and nudges the stomach upwards. They are not found in infants and are quite rare in Third World countries where diets contain more fiber and less sugar. Sliding hernias are common enough to be considered a variant of normal anatomy; Figure 3 illustrates the appearance. The drawing shows that the cardia portion of the stomach is protruding upwards through the esophageal hiatus; a slight amount is above the diaphragm and within the chest rather than the abdomen. Most people with GERD have one of these sliding hernias.

This colored surgeons' thinking and explains their fixation on the hiatal hernia in patients with GERD. The possibility of a diaphragmatic hernia of any kind was the one noted by Paré. In the early eighteenth century the famous Italian pathologist Morgagni

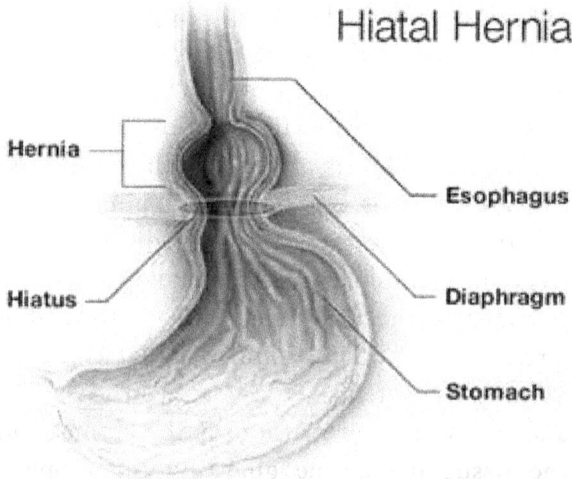

Hiatal Hernia

FIGURE 3.

identified a true hiatal hernia, apparently of the giant variety, while performing an autopsy on a man who died after protracted vomiting. As he described it, "within the thorax was found ... the stomach ... having been admitted into that cavity by the same foramen [i.e., the esophageal hiatus] through which the gula is brought down ..." During the years following, there were occasional descriptions of an autopsy finding of a hiatal hernia, usually of the large variety, but they elicited little medical attention. The proliferation of x-ray availability after William Roentgen's demonstration of his cathode ray in Paris in 1895 transformed this complacency to interest as hernias could now be diagnosed premortem. All that was required was to have the patient swallow a radiopaque liquid (barium is now the agent of choice) and the stomach and esophagus could be readily identified. As the twentieth century progressed, inevitably, as they are quite common, sliding hiatal hernias began to be detected and, because of concerns related to the potential for complications of incarceration and strangulation, surgeons began to operate to repair them.

The ability to use x-ray to image internal organs has contributed significantly to our ability to identify pathologic entities. However, in its early use, as with the case with hiatal hernias, this on occasion led clinicians astray, inducing them to treat not only benign conditions but even normal anatomy. For instance, when x-rays were taken of a standing person, the kidneys appeared lower than the anatomy books showed; their representations were based on dissections of cadavers lying supine. When upright, gravity simply allowed the normal kidneys to sag, and surgeons began to operate on patients with vague abdominal symptoms to return these "floating kidneys" to their proper location. This misinterpretation was eventually sorted out and the practice of this well-intended but futile operation ceased.

Similarly, surgeons began to repair radiologically detected hiatal hernias because they were hernias. This practice persisted through the first half of the twentieth century, although it must, or at least should, have been noticed that there were no reported instances of incarceration, much less strangulation, caused by this common hernia. Surgeons' focus began to change in response to new findings, when pathologists observed and described evidence of esophagitis during postmortem examinations. The suffix "-itis" signifies inflammation—so esophagitis is an inflammatory condition of the mucosa, the epithelium (lining) of the esophagus. Learning of its existence was a step toward understanding and identifying acid reflux disease: *something* was irritating the esophagus. Endoscopists began to identify esophagitis visually during endoscopic exams by observing a reddened discoloration, the result of stomach acid eating through the epithelium, allowing the color of the underlying blood vessels to show through. As the erosion progresses, it creates small ulcerations of the mucosa.

Of interest is the story of how the military physician William Beaumont in 1833 documented the digestive and corrosive power of stomach juices. He took advantage of a patient who survived a gunshot that created a fistula or connection between his stomach and anterior abdominal wall. Beaumont peered through this artificial aperture and could easily observe the gastric mucosa and its secretions. He learned he could affect the mucosa's appearance and the volume of gastric fluid production by varying the food he gave his patient and by stimulating mood swings. He collected the gastric secretions and poured the liquid on a variety of substances. By carefully documenting the damage done, he showed the corrosive capability of the combination of gastric acid and its digestive enzyme. When reflux occurs, this mixture is what bathes the esophagus.

It was Chevalier Jackson who, in 1929, articulated the cause of esophageal inflammation as "the retrograde flow of gastric juice." As Beaumont demonstrated, the glands of the stomach secrete a very powerful acid which contributes importantly to digestion both by its direct effects on food and by converting the pre-enzyme pepsinogen, also secreted by the gastric epithelium, into the digestive enzyme pepsin. The specialized epithelium of the stomach easily tolerates this milieu of acid and digestive enzymes and is not harmed by it. The lining of the esophagus, on the other hand, is squamous epithelium—the same as the outer layer of our skin. So, as they would be to the skin covering our bodies, these acidic gastric contents are extremely irritating, even destructive, to the lining of the esophagus.

In 1951, the British surgeon Philip Allison published his land-mark paper, "Reflux Esophagitis, Sliding Hiatal Hernia, and the Anatomy of Repair." This publication marked the tipping point. He recognized that the appropriate indication for surgical intervention was actual symptoms, not the simple presence of a hernia. His unim-provable description of a representative patient with typical symp-toms deserves unedited quotation for its accurate depiction and even a sampling of dry British wit:

> "A woman of 50 years of age complains that for 6 years she has suffered from intense burning pain behind the lower part of her sternum which rises up toward, or even into, the neck. The pain may spread into the jaw, the ear or the hard palate, or radiate through to the back between the shoulder blades, or down the arm. It comes on especially when she exerts herself stooping forward, as in washing the floor, bending over the wash tub, poking the fire, or fastening her shoes. It wakes her up in the middle of the night, especially if she is sleeping on her back or on her right side, and she seeks relief from what she describes as an agonizing pain by sitting upright and taking a few sips of water, milk, or alkaline mixture. She says that her throat usually feels dry and burning. When she swallows she may be conscious of the passage of food down the gullet, it may cause a feeling of soreness and may sometimes lodge toward the lower end of the sternum, causing pain which is immediately relieved as the *bolus* passes into the stomach. If she bends forward after a meal, food or sour fluid rises into her throat and has to be swallowed again. Her husband says that for belching she takes the first prize. Four years ago she was thought to have cholecystitis [inflammation of the gallbladder] but removal of either a normal or abnormal gallbladder did not cure her. Roentgenography of her stomach and duodenum shows no evidence of ulcer. She has tried all the advertised stomach medicines with only temporary relief and has finally been told that "the nerves of her stomach have been upset by the change of life."

"The symptoms are those of esophagitis from the reflux of gastric contents into the esophagus, due to incompetence of the gastroesophageal junction ... it is the irritation of the esophagus which causes the symptoms...."

Allison's patient manifests the typical spectrum of symptoms and a common clinical course for a patient with GERD. There is the classical heartburn, an epigastric burning pain radiating upward beneath the sternum. The typical occurrence of regurgitation of sour gastric contents into the mouth is present and associated with postures which place the *esophago*gastric junction in a dependent position. There is dysphagia, an occasional concomitant symptom, which is caused by acid irritation and disruption of esophageal muscular function. Obtaining real but fleeting relief from short lived acid neutralizers is certainly typical as is both the history of removal of the gallbladder the—incorrectly—suspected culprit and the implication that it is all in her head. The prize-winning belching results from the refluxer's tendency to frequently swallow watery saliva which is also alkaline. This is beneficial as the saliva some-what neutralizes, dilutes, and washes the refluxed acidic mate-rial into the stomach; however, air is also swallowed and belching capable of impressing spouses is the result.

The clinical community responded to this new information and supportive insights followed. In the 1920s barium was placed in patients' stomachs and gastroesophageal reflux identified radiolog-ically when it was seen to back up into the esophagus and patients experienced epigastric (upper abdominal) and/or substernal discomfort at the time the reflux occurred, i.e., they had heartburn. The quote above from Jackson shared his 1929 insight in his presen-tation, "Peptic Ulcer of the Esophagus" which reported patients with esophageal damage from, as he thought, reflux of gastric contents containing acid and pepsin. Following another similar presentation at the American Medical Society in 1934, "peptic esophagitis" entered the medical lexicon. Unfortunately, surgeons were slow to be persuaded and in the 1930s and 1940s continued to operate primarily because of enduring fixation on preventing hernia complications but with increasing appreciation of associated symptoms. The assumption persisted that the symptoms were due to the hernia.

Clinical experience and investigations such as those I was involved with in Chicago have definitively identified that the source of all symptoms is reflux through an incompetent gastroesophageal junction (or cardia or the lower esophageal sphincter). The critical issue and appropriate focus is GERD and not a hiatal hernia. Similarly, while this condition was often referred to as esophagitis, it has been clear for many years that actual inflammation of the esophagus is not always present in a symptomatic sufferer. While postmortem findings emphasized inflammatory changes, the introduction of relatively small and flexible endoscopes has allowed clinical detection of the presence or absence of esophagitis allowing us to learn that acid reflux is irritating enough to produce all the typical symptomatic manifestations without significant inflammatory changes in the mucosa.

Allison's contribution was to shift the profession's emphasis from the sliding hiatal hernia to what we now call GERD by showing that repair of the hernia did not relieve symptoms. Most people with the common hiatal hernias do not have GERD. Yet most patients with GERD do have sliding hernias. It is easy to see how surgeons were lured into mistaking the hernia as the cause of the symptoms.

Allison's carefully thought-out operation was performed through a left chest thoracotomy and was an elegant and successful procedure for anatomic repair of hiatal hernias. He successfully corrected the hernia but did nothing to reestablish an anatomic orientation of tissues that would act as a barrier to gastroesophageal reflux. To his credit, Allison did not flinch from publishing his poor results, as he acknowledged that the symptoms of GERD were not consistently or reliably controlled in his patients. He did not understand the defect was the inability to prevent acid reflux.

It also interesting that we have learned that the problem for those with GERD is not an excess amount of the acid the stomach normally produces to aid in breaking food down so that it can be further digested and absorbed in the small intestine. It would be logical to speculate that refluxers generate a large pool of stomach acid which simply overflows into the esophagus. Not the case. The amount of gastric acid in refluxers is normal. The abnormality is the loss of the ability of the lower sphincter to exert a strong enough squeeze to maintain a competent barrier guarding the esophagus from the normal acid in the stomach.

Following Allison's insight that repairing the hiatal hernia was insufficient to control symptoms, surgeons were challenged to develop a moderate number of procedures to curtail acid reflux. All to some extent wrap or fold the gastric fundus (the top part of the stomach) around the esophagus; we would describe this as a "fundo-plication," from "plicate" meaning to fold. The procedures developed by the two surgeons discussed below have dominated in the sense of being the most frequently performed. One operation was the result of a directed and sequential process, and the other a serendipitous result noticed by a prepared mind. One is most frequently performed through the abdomen: no chests are cracked. However, it is a proce-dure performed by general thoracic surgeons to protect the esoph-agus, a chest organ.

Ronald Belsey

Ronald Belsey, a British surgeon a few years younger than, and influ-enced by Allison, was a remarkably astute clinician who purpose-fully set out to develop an operation specifically to correct the underlying defect of loss of gastroesophageal competency against reflux. As you know from earlier chapters, after mandatory retire-ment from the British Health Service, he spent several months each year with us at the University of Chicago. I benefited from exposure to this remarkable man and surgeon, learning surgical techniques and absorbing stories about other surgeons of his era and of his earlier achievements.

Like all British surgeons he was addressed as "Mister" rather than "Doctor," a residual effect of the days when surgeons and barbers were considered together, and neither in the same category as

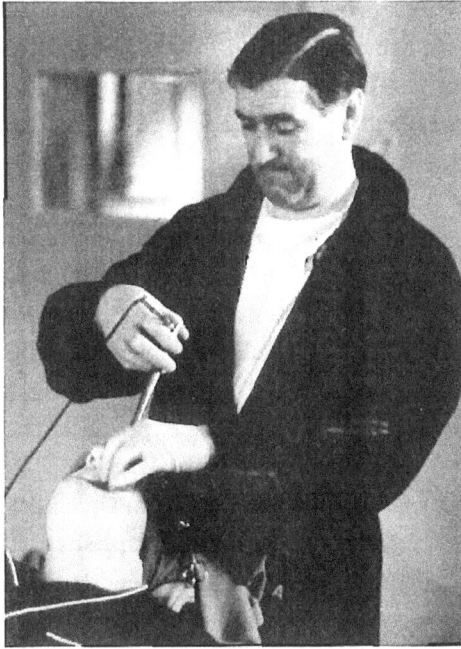

FIGURE 4.

physicians. Working in the absence of modern esophageal function testing to objectively measure acid reflux he, like a latter-day medical Sherlock Holmes, observed, listened to, and deduced insights from his experiences with patients in Bristol, England beginning in the 1940s. As he forged an antireflux operation, he combined the clinical insights he obtained with observations made during esophagoscopy, enhanced by his knowledge of anatomy and physiology.

Esophagoscopy is a procedure in which a physician inserts a viewing instrument through the mouth into the esophagus to view its mucosa. The current instrument is both flexible and considerably thinner than the scope of that time and uses fiberoptic technology to provide a magnified image on a video screen. In Figure 4, Mr. Belsey is shown in the act. He is wearing a comfortable robe to cover his surgical scrubs. As a result of his calmness and skill, augmented by a light dose of sedation, the patient, seated in a barber's chair, is apparently comfortable despite having a rigid instrument passed through his mouth and down the esophagus. The rigid scope was simply a tube which provided a direct view but with poor illumination and without magnification. Nonetheless, Belsey was patient and skilled enough to make and appreciate significant observations.

The normal cardia or gastroesophageal junction is closed except when we swallow, and it opens to let food through. In his patients, Belsey noted a gaping cardia; as the patient breathed in, expanding the chest and creating negative pressure. He further noted that gastric contents rose into the esophagus.

He pictured the requirements for an effective surgery based on his interpretation of his observations. He realized he first needed to secure the cardia below the diaphragm, well inside the abdomen. In this location, the esophagus would be exposed to the positive intra-abdominal pressure, squeezing it shut so stomach acid could not reflux up. In contrast, if the cardia were in the chest, negative pressure would keep the cardia open. He accomplished this by dissecting the esophagus within the chest so that, freed from its tissue attachments, a lengthy segment could be brought sufficiently below the diaphragm without any tendency to retract upwards.

The second thing he reasoned necessary for a successful operation was to narrow the esophageal hiatus to provide a buttress of the diaphragm against which the intra-abdominal esophagus could be compressed when the patient strained and generated positive pressure within the abdomen. Compressing the esophagus equally with the stomach would neutralize any tendency to literally squeeze gastric juices up and out. This second goal required suturing the esophageal hiatus sufficiently closed to restore its normal close proximity to the esophagus. In his inimitable words, his goal was, "the restoration of conjugal relations between the cardia and the ... [diaphragm]."

Finally, he sought to establish a valve mechanism allowing unrestricted flow of esophageal contents down into the stomach but discouraging reflux of gastric contents. He created the valve he envisioned by suturing the gastric fundus for 270 degrees around the esophagus in an inkwell fashion, causing the esophagus to enter the stomach obliquely. This partial imbrication of the esophagus resulted in a flap valve configuration. As the stomach filled and was distended, it would push closed the "flap" so acid could not gain access to the esophagus.

One of Mr. Belsey's professional attributes was his commitment to long-term follow-up of his patients so he could be sure
his results were permanent. I quote, "The battlefields of surgery
are strewn with the remains of promising new operations which
perished in the follow-up clinic." (He stressed this point when
we operated together. A surgeon isn't successful just because the
patient survived the operation—the goal is a high quality for the
remainder of the patient's life.) This was coupled with his enviable
ability to be self-critical, and not let ego deter him from an honest
appraisal of the results of his procedure, a challenging characteristic to emulate. Accordingly, when he was unsatisfied with the
status of his early patients, he modified the operation, all the while
keeping his surgical principles in mind.

Using a British system of nomenclature, he progressed from
the initial version called the Mark I through two subsequent itera-
tions before arriving at the final version, the Belsey Mark IV operation. The final result was much more complex than a simple hernia
repair. Operating through the left chest, the esophagus and stomach
were significantly rearranged to restore as near as possible the
conditions of normal anatomy and physiology that protect against
acid reflux but permit belching so that excess gastric bloating after
eating did not occur.

Figures 5A and 5B illustrate his procedure. A side view of a
Belsey Mark IV operation is shown in Figure 5A. On the left is
depicted the placement of sutures from the esophagus to the
stomach which return through the diaphragm to the esophagus.
The rightmost drawing in Figure 5A shows the appearance after
the sutures are tied. The result is a rolling up of the stomach around
the esophagus. Both organs are firmly anchored to the diaphragm,
reducing the chances of development of a postoperative hiatal
hernia. The drawing on the left in Figure 5B is a side view of the
final appearance of the operation. The x-ray on the right with
barium in the stomach illustrates how this angulates the esophageal entry into the stomach. This configuration creates a flap valve
which results in the esophagus being compressed shut when the
stomach is distended, for example after a meal, thus deterring acid
reflux.

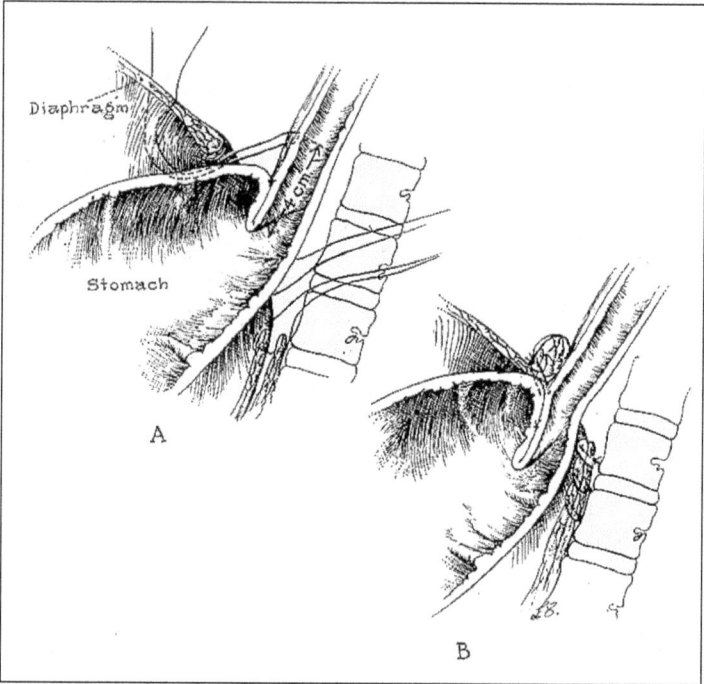

Diaphragm

Stomach

A

B

FIGURE 5A.

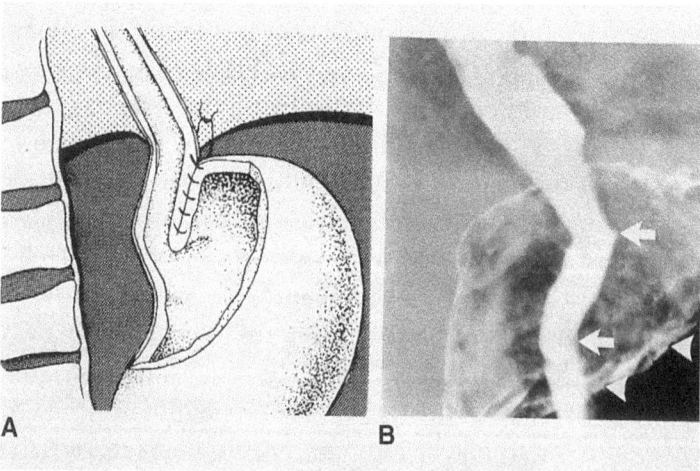

A

B

FIGURE 5B.

He continued to follow the cohort of his patients who were treated with the Mark IV procedure to be certain his good early results stood the test of time. The following quote illustrates his appreciation that surgery for a benign and functional disorder required more than the patient surviving the operation. "Whereas mortality rates are of greater interest to the surgeon, who fosters the illusion that his value to society is judged largely by the number of patients he does, or does not, slaughter; to the patient the question of how prolonged will be the period of post-operative misery is of far greater moment than any consideration of immortality."

Mr. Belsey waited until 1967, having compiled several decades of experience with his operation and the follow-up of his patients, to inform the thoracic surgery community of its benefits by presenting his experience at the annual meeting of the prestigious American Association for Thoracic Surgery and subsequently publishing the seminal article, "The Surgical Management of Esophageal Reflux and Hiatus Hernia." Despite the fact that many of his patients began with severe reflux with esophageal damage including active inflammation and strictures (scarring due to healing of erosive esophagitis), fully 85% of his patients had no further GERD symptoms and most of the remaining patients were improved. These results would still be acceptable today. Even further, in addition to describing the Mark IV procedure, in the article he examined the pathophysiology of GERD and detailed the pertinent clinical aspects of the typical patient. Of note, he only finally allowed airing of his technique and results after sufficient follow-up had been achieved, and at the behest of David Skinner. Skinner, my University of Chicago mentor, at that time was a surgical resident based in Boston spending several months training in England. He and Belsey bonded to the extent that Skinner reviewed Belsey's carefully compiled patient records and was actually listed as first author of the article describing the Mark IV procedure.

Belsey produced this achievement while working in Bristol in a modest-sized hospital in the southwest of England with no connection to a medical school. Here he performed both adult and pediatric cardiac surgery, as well as esophageal and lung surgery. His rural, semi-isolated lifestyle fit his personality perfectly. He was an enthusiastic outdoorsman, lived on a working farm, and enjoyed salmon fishing on the river that meandered through his property. The environment also fit his professional life: he was fully self-reliant and had no interest in participating in the political jostlings of the British academic surgical community centered in London. He was not always alone, however. Because of his reputation as a surgeon par excellence and connections made as a research fellow at the Massachusetts General Hospital, he trained and mentored a constant stream of surgery residents from prestigious institutions around the world, including Johns Hopkins, Massachusetts General Hospital, several European centers, and other international locations. He proved to be a patient and thoughtful teacher, and many of his trainees went on to be leaders of thoracic surgery both in the USA and across Europe. As a result, the Belsey School continues to exert a significant impact on the international practice of thoracic surgery. I can speak firsthand of his technical prowess, teaching skills, and personal magnetism.

Rudolph Nissen

Nissen's life story is a remarkable testament to perseverance and grace under pressure. He was born in Germany, where he proved to be a superior student and eventually a talented surgeon. His skills and work ethic resulted in his becoming a protégée of Sauerbruch, the leader of German surgery mentioned in Chapter Six. This is the same man who developed the negative pressure operating chamber to prevent lung collapse during intrathoracic surgery. Being Sauerbruch's associate was a stepping-stone to a successful career in academic surgery in Germany. However, as a Jew, Nissen became increasingly uncomfortable with Hitler's programs and the anti-Semitic atmosphere that prevailed in Germany. His tolerance at an end, he began a peripatetic life, departing Germany in 1933 to assume the Chair of the Department of Surgery at the University of Istanbul, later observing, "I am glad that I left Germany ... which saved me from witnessing firsthand the weakness of character that a majority of university professors exhibited at the time." His surgical skills and personal attributes made him a success in Istanbul; no less a person than Kemal Atatürk was a patient.

Unfortunately, continued harassment by the National Socialists through the German Embassy continued to make life precarious for him and his family, so he relocated again, this time to the USA. With remarkable patience, perseverance, and humility, he began as a research assistant and worked to establish himself anew. He thrived and, literally, carved out yet another successful career, eventually practicing in New York and Boston from 1939 until 1952. Nissen operated on Einstein in 1948, wrapping his abdominal aortic aneurysm with cellophane, the standard procedure of the day. This staved off the inevitable fatal rupture for another seven years. (Today, the weakened and abnormally dilated aorta would be replaced with a tubular graft, and normal life expectancy restored. One wonders what contributions by Einstein were lost.) In 1952, Nissen accepted his final position as Chair of the Department of Surgery at the University of Basel, Switzerland.

It was during his tenure in Istanbul that he unintentionally entered the arena of surgery for GERD. In 1937, he operated through the left chest of a 28-year-old man who had a perforated ulcer of the esophagus near the gastric junction. Nissen resected the terminal portion of the esophagus harboring the ulcer and a small amount of stomach, essentially the cardia. To restore continuity, he anastomosed (connected by sewing together) the end of the esophagus to the side of the gastric fundus. To bolster this connection, he then wrapped the relatively voluminous fundus of the stomach around the esophagus so that the anastomosis nestled within a protective cocoon, a fundoplication.

The next piece of the puzzle fell into place nearly a decade later when a patient in New York refused the standard thoracotomy approach for repair of a giant—not sliding—hiatal hernia. At that time, surgeons preferred to operate on these hernias through the chest. It is safer to push the herniated stomach back into the abdomen than pull it down from below the diaphragm as it can tear if it has become adherent to other tissue. Also, surgeons can cut tissue away to allow the esophagus sufficient mobility that it can easily be slid into the abdomen. His patient's insistence forced Nissen to operate through the abdomen. He removed the stomach from the hernia sac, returned it back into the abdominal cavity and created a gastropexy (to "*-pexy*" is to surgically fix in place) by suturing the stomach to the abdominal wall to hold the cardia and esophagus below the diaphragm, in the abdomen. He repeated this operation several times over the subsequent years—thoracotomies, and the associated pain, have never been popular with patients—and his patients did well. Specifically, he observed they did not develop heartburn or begin to regurgitate, the two hallmarks of GERD.

He completed the GERD puzzle when he returned to Europe. Nissen had the opportunity to examine the man on whom he had performed a fundoplication in 1937, and found him to be thriving, with neither clinical manifestations of GERD nor endoscopic evidence of esophagitis. His prepared mind recognized the salutary benefits of these two operations: a fundoplication in the young man and the fixation of the gastroesophageal junction in the abdomen in the patients with giant hiatal hernias. He put his insight to use in 1954 when he began to perform elective operations specifically for GERD. He started by combining a fundoplication and a gastropexy in the same operation, most frequently through the abdomen but occasionally using a chest approach.

He eventually found sewing the stomach to the undersurface of the abdominal wall, the gastropexy, was not necessary and could be omitted. The fundoplication alone, wrapping the fundus of the stomach around the esophagus, controlled reflux symptoms. For those interested in surgical details, the operation as performed today—some technical details have evolved since Nissen's time—is depicted in Figures 6A, 6B, and 6C. Figure 6A depicts the operative appearance after the surgeon has separated the distal esophagus and the gastric fundus from normal tissue attachments so that they can easily be moved and reoriented. Sutures are placed in the esophageal hiatus behind the cardia. In Figure 6B, the sutures in the hiatus have been tied to bring the muscles of the diaphragm together so that the stomach can't sneak up into the hiatus post-operatively. The gastric fundus has been pushed from the patient's left side beneath the esophagus and sutures placed to connect the stomach on the left side to the portion on the right side. In Figure 6C, the operation is complete. The gastric fundus has been wrapped

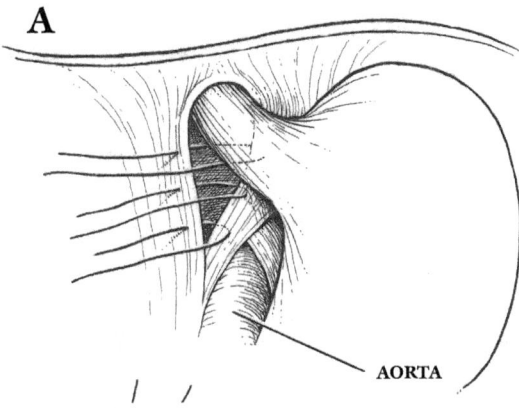

A

AORTA

FIGURE 6A.

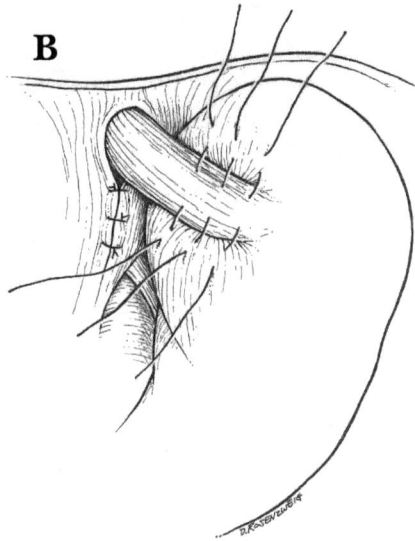

B

FIGURE 6B.

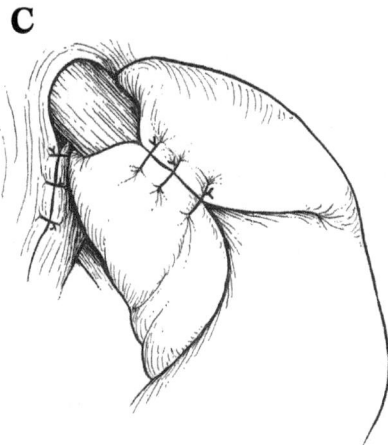

C

FIGURE 6C.

around the esophagus by tying the sutures shown in Figure 6B. The Nissen fundoplication has remained the mainstay of surgical therapy for GERD.

Studying Figures 5 and 6 to appreciate how the surgeon must reorient the stomach, esophagus, and diaphragm gives an idea of the degree of difficulty surgeons have historically encountered in solving GERD. Those curious to see the process in action can find video clips of both the Nissen and Belsey procedures on the Internet.

Current Status of Antireflux Surgery

The Belsey and Nissen operations remain by far the most frequently performed operations for GERD. Both either diminish or, usually, eliminate acid reflux. Belsey's operation causes fewer side effects, perhaps because the stomach is wrapped only 270 degrees around the esophagus compared to a complete 360-degree wrap for the Nissen. This results in more patients retaining the ability to belch than is the case for the Nissen operation. This seemingly trivial act is important in preventing excess distension of the stomach when swallowed air is trapped inside causing a quite distressing bloating sensation.

Despite this advantage, Nissen's operation has gained in popularity with surgeons for several reasons. First, Belsey's operation is technically more challenging to perform as it requires suturing the stomach directly to the esophagus which has only a thin wall of fragile muscle to which stitches must be anchored, making them at risk of pulling out over time. For the Nissen fundoplication, the thick-walled and sturdily muscled stomach is sutured to itself. (The stomach needs those strong muscles to massage its contents and break them down for absorption in the small intestine.) Secondly, although occasionally performed through the chest, Nissen and others showed that his procedure could be done through a laparotomy, an incision in the abdomen, between the bottom of the sternum and the navel. This open laparotomy causes less pain than a thoracotomy, the only approach through which a Belsey procedure is possible.

The advent of the now routine so-called minimally invasive laparoscopic approach has lessened postoperative pain even further and resulted in the patient recovering more quickly. (The techniques utilized in the performance of minimally invasive operations are discussed in the final chapter.) Over time and with experience, two modifications have been introduced which reduce the incidence of uncomfortable gas bloating with the Nissen fundoplication without diminishing its antireflux properties: the recommended length of the gastric wrap has been shortened to only two centimeters, and great importance is now placed on keeping the wrap loose around the esophagus rather than tightening it down. Although difficulty in belching remains a common side effect of the operation, the incidence of severe bloating has greatly diminished, and with some care on the patient's part to avoid overeating, it is a much less troublesome problem.

How do these operations work? As we helped to understand by our research efforts in Chicago, multiple factors are involved. Clearly, maintaining the terminal esophagus inside the positive pressure environment of the abdomen helps and is the normal anatomic situation. Any straining which constricts abdominal muscles and increases abdominal pressure tends to squeeze the stomach and extrude gastric juices up into the esophagus. However, if the squeeze is equally applied to the esophagus, the net effect is the forces cancel each other out and no reflux occurs. (An interesting corroboration of this assertion is found in the animal kingdom. The sloth spends much of its life upside down and also has a quite long abdominal component of its esophagus, presumably to prevent constant gastro-esophageal reflux.) The flap valve configuration formed by an oblique entry of the esophagus into the stomach, as discussed above, is a factor. The lower esophageal sphincter pressure is significantly lower in patients with reflux than in people without. All antireflux operations wrap the stomach around the esophagus, resulting in an increased pressure of the sphincter when measured by a motility study; this makes the sphincter more resistant to reflux. This is a result of the squeeze exerted by the gastric muscle. Restoring this pressure appears to be critical to obtaining a satisfactory outcome.

I had performed several hundred thoracic and abdominal open antireflux operations over the years by the time minimally invasive surgery made its appearance. Over the same period new and more effective drugs became available for the medical treatment of acid reflux. Both changes affected my performance of these operations in numerous ways.

Initially, I performed these operations through a laparotomy or thoracotomy, mainly for intractable heartburn. Medications to reduce acid secretion were quite helpful but did not suffice for all. Minimally invasive operation entered the general surgery realm when laparoscopic cholecystectomy (gallbladder removal) was introduced. Diehard, conservative surgeons were first appalled and even amused at the very idea "of operating through a tube." All soon had to abandon their resistance as it became a routine operation, and the first choice of patients.

I was amazed when pioneer surgeons developed and introduced minimally invasive, laparoscopic, Nissen fundoplications. Nonetheless, I had to adapt. This was my first use of laparoscopy and learning was stressful. The optics are magnificent, thanks to magnification but mastering the new instruments took time and I missed the tactile feedback from my hands and fingers to which I was accustomed.

It was worth it, however, as laparoscopic surgery performed using small abdominal incisions and video control shortened the time the patient needed to stay in the hospital, diminished postoperative pain, hastened return to normal activities, and is associated with minimal morbidity and vanishingly small mortality rates. At about the same time as this shift in antireflux surgery, a new class of drugs to suppress acid was introduced. These proton pump inhibitors (acid is the result of hydrogen ions which are single protons) are able to completely eliminate acid secretion so they are quite effective in eliminating heartburn. These surgical and medical advances had an impact on patients. Because the "new" operation is less painful and recovery is expedited, patients are more willing to undergo a procedure. But because the medications are more effective, fewer patients had uncontrollable heartburn.

My experience is representative. After I performed an open Nissen procedure through a true laparotomy, my patients usually went home a few days following their operation, required pain medication for a few weeks, and were not able to resume full activities for a month to six weeks. In contrast, when I performed a laparoscopic

Nissen fundoplication, patients went home the following day, most needed only non-narcotic analgesic medications for any lingering discomfort from the small incisions or shoulder discomfort (more about the latter to come) and could resume routine activities within a week.

Nissen fundoplication was one of my favorite operations, both open and especially laparoscopic. The risk of serious complications was nearly zero and the great majority of patients were genuinely delighted with their new life. Being rid of some combination of frequent heartburn, regurgitation, and the requirement to modify their lifestyle (including avoiding coffee, tea, chocolate, and alcohol) and take daily medications greatly improved their quality of life.

It must be remembered, however, that some heartburn is very common; experiencing it occasionally is not a disease and does not constitute a reason for surgery. In fact, not even all patients with true GERD should have an operation; it is appropriate only for the minority. Having mild or controllable heartburn does not qualify. Patients who do not achieve satisfactory relief of persistent and severe symptoms with medical management are definitely candidates.

A more controversial indication is for patients whose heartburn is reasonably controlled but who continue to regurgitate gastric contents. Medications can alter the composition of gastric contents by reducing or even eliminating the acid component but the tendency to reflux and regurgitate remains as the incompetent gastroesophageal junction is unchanged. This is not just unpleasant, but a potentially dangerous event as regurgitated gastric juice can be aspirated into the lungs and cause pneumonia.

Finally, there are patients who choose an operation for lifestyle reasons. They don't want to take medications for many years and wish—reasonably—to be able to enjoy, on a moderate basis, foods that worsen their acid reflux by weakening the muscle at the lower esophageal sphincter. This includes caffeine-containing drinks such as coffee and tea, as well as chocolate and alcohol. Since the operation is performed to enhance the quality of life, this seems to me a valid consideration as long as the procedure is safe and effective.

My experience suggests that the most common cause of unhappy patients is less a difference in surgical skills than in patient selection, being careful to only operate on the "right" patients. This means being sure the patient's quality of life is sufficiently impaired to warrant an operation and having full confidence that GERD is the correct diagnosis. I stress that mildly annoying, occasional, and easily treatable heartburn is not a sufficient indication for an operation. If there is any doubt acid reflux is the problem, both esophageal manometry and pH monitoring should be performed to be sure what's troubling the patient is not something else like achalasia, heart disease, cholecystitis (gallbladder inflammation from gallstones), or anything else. An antireflux operation in these patients will fail to help and may even worsen their condition. This challenge of properly selecting patients for surgical care was really the point of my research at the University of Chicago; measuring the amount of acid reflux is definitive. I disagree with some surgeons who espouse pH monitoring in all patients before performing antireflux surgery; however, this test should be performed if there is any question about the diagnosis. Testing the patient with symptoms, including pain and dysphagia, after an operation can help to sort things out by determining how successfully the procedure stopped reflux; if there is none, a search for other causes can begin.

Nonetheless, the pursuit of even better interventions, in varying stages of use or development, continues. One is called an "endoscopic fundoplication." During an endoscopic procedure, the endoscopist exerts traction to push the end of the esophagus down into the stomach and a device is used to staple the esophagus in that position. The final result looks somewhat like a Nissen fundoplication. Surgical innovators have also developed a magnetized metallic ring which is placed laparoscopically around the distal esophagus. The constriction it produces retards reflux, but arriving food is able to push through the magnetic attractions. Until one of these two, or some other innovation, proves itself, the laparoscopic Nissen procedure stands as the gold standard of surgical therapy for GERD.

10
▼

SURGERY FOR
ACHALASIA

E ating and breathing. Essential to life, no conscious thought or effort necessary. But there are differences between them: breathing is essential but not actually fun. Eating, if you're like me, is undeniably one of life's pleasures. Imagine what it would do to your health and morale to have to struggle to swallow, and to be unable to get food into your stomach. Everything sticks and refuses to move on down. Function is the issue, not anatomy.

This is the dispiriting state of affairs for patients with the rare motility disorder called "achalasia." As elaborated in Appendix Three, the normal sequence of events when eating is that we prepare food to be swallowed from the mouth by chewing to break it down into manageable bits while mixing them with saliva to lubricate the morsels. For the food bolus to leave the mouth, it is necessary for the upper esophageal sphincter to relax to allow it to pass from the mouth into the esophagus. The swallow stimulates the esophagus and initiates a wave of sequential esophageal contractions—called "peristalsis"—that propel the food down the esophagus toward the stomach. When the food bolus reaches the lower esophagus, it encounters the lower sphincter which relaxes to permit passage into the stomach.

Every aspect of esophageal function is deranged in achalasia, a disease of unknown etiology which causes two primary symptoms. Dysphagia is the predominant one, usually starting in a person's teenage years. The difficulty swallowing is typically mild and intermittent at its onset; just a nuisance. As the patient ages the severity of the difficulty in getting food through the esophagus worsens. Affected individuals have no difficulty in the first phase of swallowing; they can clear their mouth without difficulty. The problem begins when the food enters the esophagus. Patients are arguably worse off than the mythological Tantalus, who was exposed to food and water which retreated beyond his grasp as he reached for them, giving rise to our modern term, "tantalizing." Those with achalasia can reach food, put it in their mouth and then begin to swallow, but once the food is in the esophagus its progress comes to a halt. Liquids may trickle through the esophagus but as the sufferer ages, it becomes progressively more difficult and eventually impossible to complete the swallowing process with solid foods, no matter how well chewed. Concomitantly with the worsening dysphagia, the second symptom the patient experiences is regurgitation. Regurgitation is a passive phenomenon; esophageal contents accumulating in the esophagus simply spill out into the mouth when the patient bends over or lies flat. This can be contrasted to vomiting, an active process caused by contractions of the stomach which forcibly propel gastric contents up and out. They are at risk of developing pneumonia if the regurgitated food is aspirated into the trachea. An awake person would simply cough out any material that was aspirated. However, if regurgitation and aspiration take place during sleep, the material can easily contaminate the lungs and lead to the development of pneumonia. The cumulative effect of the regurgitation and difficulty swallowing is weight loss, sometimes to the point of emaciation.

The typical major complaint by a patient to a physician is a history of dysphagia which began as a mild nuisance, typically in the second or third decade of life, and has progressively worsened, particularly for solid foods. This suggests the diagnosis as young patients are unlikely to have esophageal cancer, another cause of esophageal obstruction. The appearance of an enlarged esophagus with a narrowing at its terminal end on a barium contrast x-ray (but without a mass as is seen in patients with esophageal cancer) further strengthens the likelihood of achalasia. However, an esophageal motility study is necessary to definitively pin down the diagnosis. Even without this study we can be reasonably certain that achalasia has been a disrupter of esophageal function and the quality of patients' lives for many years.

An early encounter with achalasia probably occurred in 1674 when an ingenious physician named Thomas Willis in England reported his interaction with a patient with "food blockage in [his] esophagus." Without any clinical tests to guide him, Willis was limited to the patient's description of his inability to get food into his stomach. He regurgitated most of what he swallowed. He could clear his mouth, but the food remained in the esophagus. He was clearly malnourished. Willis concluded, "The mouth of the stomach [the cardia] being always closed either by a tumor or palsie, nothing could be admitted into the ventricle [stomach] unless it were violently opened." Willis took a whale's rib (something the prepared physician of the day apparently kept on hand), wrapped its tip with a sponge and had the patient pass this device through his mouth, exactly as a sword swallower would do, and push the food which had collected in the lower esophagus past the lower esophageal sphincter and into the stomach. His description, with its idiosyncratic use of capitals, common for the time, of his patient's ability to tolerate this unique treatment:

"No less will a very rare case of a certain Man of Oxford shew an almost perpetual Vomiting to be stirred up by the shutting up of the left orifice [the cardia]. A strong Man, and otherwise healthful enough, labouring for a long time with often Vomiting, he was wont … to cast up whatsoever he had eaten. At length the Disease having overcome all remedies, he was brought into that condition, that growing hungry he would eat until the Oesophagus was filled up to the Throat, in the mean time nothing sliding down into the Ventricle [stomach], he cast up raw whatsoever he had taken in … and he languished from hunger and every day was in danger of Death. I prepared an instrument for him like a Rod, of whale Bone with a little round Button of Sponge fixed to the top of it; the sick man having taken down meat and drink into his Throat, presently putting it down the Oesophagus he did thrust down into the ventricle ... the Food which otherwise would have come back again; and by this means he hath daily taken sustenance for 15 years ... who would otherwise perish for want of Food."

This maneuvering with the whale bone plunger kept the man from starving to death but we might imagine he encountered some difficulty in retaining dinner companions. We also can have confidence in the achalasia diagnosis as the cause of his dysphagia. Cancer would have quickly done him in, and a stricture—scarring inside the esophagus caused by severe acid reflux—would not have responded so well to the whale bone regimen.

Johann von Mikulicz, who, during his career often moved within the region that is now Austria, Poland, and Germany, was an influential surgeon with multiple contributions to surgery to his credit. Those particularly relevant to thoracic surgery include the mentoring of Sauerbruch with whom he worked to develop the negative pressure chamber for thoracic surgical procedures, and the invention of one of the first endoscopes physicians used to view the interior of the esophagus and stomach. He used his invention in 1881 on a patient who was unable to swallow normally and noted that the cardia did not relax and open spontaneously to expose the stomach as he had observed in other patients. He astutely called this observed phenomenon "cardiospasm," suggesting an inappropriate muscular squeeze. Mikulicz finally acted on his interpretation 23 years later in 1904—probably with the next patient he encountered with this rare disorder—and successfully treated him by inserting a finger up into his esophagus through an incision he made in the stomach and forcibly stretching open the cardia musculature.

His renown for this and his many other accomplishments resulted in Mikulicz being frequently invited to consult on distant patients. As related by Laskowski, one experience resulted in a remarkable display of hospitality. "On one such trip, Mikulicz relieved the phimosis (a narrowing of the foreskin) of the son of a nobleman. [Not all operations are glamorous.] After the successful procedure, the surgeon was feted at a banquet in his honor. By the middle of the night, only half the courses had been served and Mikulicz felt satiated, but on the stroke of midnight, 12 barbers with assistants entered, shaved their guests, and refreshed them with hot and cold compresses and then withdrew for the banquet to continue." Laskowski concludes, "Times were indeed different then." Seems like an event for which Downton Abbey would be the perfect setting. I can see Carson the butler orchestrating the proceedings.

The anatomical site of the dysfunction, if not the cause, in patients with achalasia located, surgeons began to do what their first instincts usually tell them to do—cut something out. A small number of operations to resect, to actually remove, the cardia were performed in Europe. The results were not good. There were significant complications, particularly leakage of stomach contents through the anastomosis rejoining the esophagus to the stomach when it did not heal properly. These surgeons were fixated on the anatomy of the problem; what was required was the ability to think of and direct action toward the malfunctioning of the esophagus.

This step was taken in 1913 by the German surgeon Ernst Heller, who performed the first operative procedure that did not require actually removing the offending gastroesophageal junction. He dissected his patient's esophagus free from surrounding tissue through an abdominal approach. He carefully preserved the inner mucosal layer as he cut the overlying muscle longitudinally on two sides, which is called a "*myo*tomy." He extended the incisions from the esophagus across the cardia and on to the stomach to create a double myotomy operation for achalasia. There were two cuts of the esophageal and gastric muscle, both of which cross the esophago-gastric junction, the location of the non-relaxing lower esophageal sphincter. This double esophagomyotomy successfully lowered the pressure in the sphincter sufficiently to diminish its resistance to the passage of food and improve his patients' ability to eat and swallow.

A few years after Heller introduced his operation, the medical community named this disorder "achalasia," a name derived by combining the prefix *a* signifying "non-" with the Greek *chalasis*, meaning slackening or relaxing. This emphasized that the abnormality was a failure of relaxation of the cardia or lower esophageal sphincter. Even though this understanding gradually sank in, Heller's technique was not immediately adopted by other surgeons. Although resectional operations with their complications were abandoned, surgeons used a variety of procedures, all of which widened the cardia (for example, with a longitudinal incision which was closed transversely, thus making the cardia shorter but wider). While these operations lessened dysphagia and improved the ability to swallow, many patients complained of unrelenting and excruciating heartburn. The cause was florid acid reflux from the stomach through the surgically widened cardia. It did not take long for surgeons to abandon these operations.

Eventually, by the middle of the last century, Heller's approach had become the standard operation, although with some modifications. Surgeons preferred to use a left thoracotomy for the operation and this approach supplanted the abdominal approach. Experience showed that using the chest to operate on the esophagus and cardia was associated with less postoperative reflux, probably because it required less dissection of the hiatus, thus preserving a modicum of the native antireflux anatomy. Surgeons also quickly learned that performing only a single myotomy was sufficient. Because of the concern over postoperative reflux there was a debate over the advisability of adding an antireflux procedure to the myotomy, as weakening the cardia clearly enables some reflux to occur, even if less than following an abdominal operation.

This is the operation I learned in Chicago during my residency. A left thoracotomy is used and a myotomy is begun on the esophagus and extended across the cardia and onto the stomach. The antireflux procedure Belsey developed completes the operation. The Belsey addendum to the myotomy, while diminishing the likelihood of postoperative acid reflux, does not increase the lower esophageal sphincter pressure as much as the Nissen procedure, so it does not interfere with the passage of food through the gastroesophageal junction. (The surgeon doesn't want to surgically re-create the same difficulty swallowing for which the operation was indicated.) I performed this operation for many years before it was overtaken by the revolution of minimally invasive surgical techniques. After some initial skepticism, the laparoscopic technique was eventually shown to be superior to a thoracoscopic approach and is the current surgical method of choice. All the technical requirements for a satisfactory operation can be met, most importantly that of an adequate myotomy (a single myotomy is sufficient but it must cross the gastroesophageal junction) to significantly lower the resting pressure of the lower esophageal sphincter. An antireflux operation can be added to reduce the severity of postoperative reflux although it must not reobstruct the gastroesophageal junction.

These requirements rule out the use of the Nissen procedure with its complete wrap of the stomach around the esophagus. There are several ways to create partial wraps which resemble the Belsey procedure that can be used instead. This laparoscopic operation gives at least 90% of patients an improved ability to swallow. Swallowing is restored to nearly normal (rarely completely to normal as explained below) and patients experience no or only mild acid reflux, and heartburn which can be easily treated with antacids or acid suppression medications.

Motility studies such as the ones we performed at the University of Chicago have identified the abnormalities of esophageal function associated with achalasia. While the lower esophageal sphincter pressure is found to be elevated in some patients, the pressure is typically within the range of normal. The consistent abnormality of the sphincter is that it does not relax with a swallow as it should, so swallowed food encounters a closed sphincter. Mikulicz was on the right track; however, there is no "spasm," a term which implies a strong squeeze and a higher than normal pressure.

An unexpected concomitant abnormality is that the esophageal body affected by achalasia no longer has the ability to propel food; there is a complete loss of peristalsis. The esophageal contractions are typically weaker than normal and, most importantly, occur simultaneously, not sequentially, so they are unable to propel a bolus of food through the lower sphincter. These findings explain the patient's symptoms. The only way for food to get into the stomach is for a food column to build high enough in the esophagus for the pressure at the bottom to exceed the sphincter pressure.

I picture something similar to a geologist's view of earth's strata; a layer of breakfast sitting on top of the preceding dinner on top of lunch on top of yesterday's breakfast which is finally forced into the stomach by the weight of the column of food. As the food piles up, it inexorably stretches and enlarges the body of the tubular esophagus. The vivid mental picture of this capacious esophagus full to the brim of food explains why regurgitation of the top stratum into the mouth is also a symptom of achalasia. When the patient bends over or stoops, the highest food layer is close to the top of the esophagus and simply spills out into the mouth. This derangement in esophageal motility is responsible for the inability of an operation to render a patient's swallowing completely normal; the operation cannot affect the body of the esophagus. There is less resistance to the passage of food at the lower sphincter but without peristalsis some food may sit in the flaccid esophagus until it is emptied by gravity.

As with antireflux operations, the laparoscopic procedure gets patients out of the hospital sooner than either a thoracotomy or a laparotomy and is associated with less pain and a quicker recovery to normal activity. Nearly all patients are significantly improved by the combination of laparoscopic myotomy and the appropriate antireflux procedure. They can eat most solid foods and both the severity and frequency of regurgitation decrease. However, prudence in eating is encouraged as they are not returned to normal in their ability to get food down. This is an early challenge for patients who may not have enjoyed solid food for years and want to hit the first buffet they can find. It's true—the myotomy decreases the lower sphincter pressure and food has an easier time passing through but without sequential contractions to sweep food along, emptying of the esophagus is dependent on gravity. Consequently, there remains a tendency for the inefficient esophagus to retain some swallowed material, particularly if the eager patient eats too rapidly, so the possibility of regurgitation and aspiration, though much reduced, remains.

Though we have this safe, effective and minimally invasive operation, the search for even better interventions continues. There is early experience with an endoscopic technique which begins with passing an endoscopic instrument into the esophagus. An incision is made in the esophageal lining, the mucosa. The endoscope is then snaked through the incision and into the anatomic plane between the mucosa and the muscle. The esophageal muscle is incised downward from this point until the muscle constituting the lower sphincter has been divided, much like the standard surgical myotomy. The mucosal defect is stapled shut from inside after the scope is withdrawn. Spending a lifetime dreading leaks of esophageal contents into the chest or abdomen, caused by traumatic injuries or the failure of a surgical anastomosis, which are typically devastating as they leak bacteria-laden saliva or food into the chest, has made me nervous about this technique. However, the early results are encouraging, and patients will flock to this alternative if it proves itself, as it requires no external incision and leaves no scars. (Laparoscopy requires five incisions, none of which are longer than a centimeter and quickly blend into normal skin creases as they heal.) Perhaps this will one day be the standard procedure.

There are non-surgical therapies available but all have drawbacks. There are medications such as nitroglycerine and calcium channel blockers which relax smooth muscle, but they don't sufficiently weaken the lower esophageal sphincter to significantly reduce the impediment to the passage of food and are associated with unpleasant side effects such as headache. Dilation—stretching the cardia from the inside during an endoscopy—has some success; however, as gentle stretching is insufficient, it must be done by the rapid inflation of a balloon (the procedure is called "pneumatic dilation") inside the esophagus, straddling the lower esophageal sphincter, with sufficient vigor to actually rupture the muscle. There are occasional full-thickness tears of the esophagus, actual perforations, which require emergency surgery to repair. In addition, the long-term success rate for dilation of satisfactorily improved swallowing is less than for an operative myotomy.

Botulinum toxin (the same Botox used to smooth out facial wrinkles) can be injected into the muscle at the cardia through an endoscope. This is effective as it relaxes the muscle and improves the patient's ability to swallow but the results are not durable: the effect wears off as the toxin is metabolized, and the procedure must be repeated every few months. Botox injections seem not to impair the ability to perform a surgical myotomy—unless used with excess frequency which can cause inflammatory scarring obliterating the space between the muscle and the mucosa. If the muscle is welded to the mucosa, the surgeon cannot incise the muscle without also cutting the mucosa, thus creating a full-thickness defect in the esophageal wall. Botox injections can be used judiciously to allow the patient temporary relief while planning for the operation at their convenience. Since the laparoscopic procedure is effective, safe, has replaced a painful thoracotomy, and has shortened the length of hospitalization, the pendulum has swung toward minimally invasive surgical therapy as the first choice for most patients.

An unsolved question is the cause of achalasia. In the early eighteenth century some in the medical community, perhaps premature Freudians, explained difficulty swallowing as being caused by "irrational love" or "uncontrolled desires." Although it seems safe to rule these causes out, no definitive etiology (cause or origin) for achalasia has been identified. Some patients recall their mothers identifying excessive childhood regurgitation, but most become aware of the onset of difficulty getting food all the way down as teenagers or in their twenties, when they usually begin to seek medical care. Yet the onset is rarely at birth, suggesting the disease is acquired and not congenital. Possible etiologies include a degenerative process (there are fewer normal intrinsic nerves in the wall of the esophagus than usual, suggesting they have been destroyed); an autoimmune phenomenon (a substantial number of patients do have detectable antibodies to esophageal nerves); or an infectious disease. A clue may come from Chagas's disease, an infectious process found primarily in Latin America, which causes difficulty swallowing and is identical to achalasia as regards the derangements of esophageal function. It is the result of an infection with the parasite *Trypanosoma cruzi*. While there is some evidence for each one of these three mechanisms (as well as for all three together, as an infection can trigger an autoimmune process which results in nerve degeneration), the true cause of achalasia remains a mystery.

As the minimally invasive rising tide scooped up operations for achalasia, I abandoned the old (open thoracotomy) for the new (laparoscopy). My patient AC was in his mid-twenties and what had begun in his teen years with the occasional sense of food sticking on the way down had become almost complete inability to swallow solid food. In addition, he occasionally regurgitated bits of chewed but undigested particles of his meals and had gotten through one bout of pneumonia. Not surprisingly, he was thin. He was nervous about my recommendation of surgery but knew he needed relief.

In the operating room I placed AC supine (flat on his back) with his legs suspended in stirrups so I could stand between his legs. I inserted five ports, retracted the liver from view and began the process of separating the esophagus from the hiatus. When I had fully exposed it, I made a small cut through the muscle of the anterior surface. Aided by the video magnification, I could now easily distinguish the mucosal lining that needed to be protected from the overlying muscle. I extended the cut in the muscle up the esophagus and down onto the stomach. This was to be sure all the muscle fibers that constitute the lower esophageal sphincter were fully divided; this is the sine qua non of the operation. To minimize acid reflux later in life, I folded the fundus of the stomach over the myotomy and sutured it in this configuration; this Toupet procedure diminishes reflux without compromising swallowing.

AC recovered uneventfully and two weeks after his operation he could eat anything but confessed that if he bolted something without sufficient chewing it might stick for several minutes until he could wash it down. So, as is typical, his swallowing was improved but not fully normal. He also experienced one of the major benefits of a laparoscopic operation—not enough pain to ever require narcotics for relief.

11

▼

HEADING WEST

I nevitably, as time passed, there were changes within the Chicago
Department of Surgery. After my first three years on the faculty,
DeMeester departed to become chair of another department of
surgery. I was given the opportunity to move into his vacated slot as
Chief of the Division of Thoracic Surgery. This began my involvement with medical school administration, and meant I was now
responsible for organizing and directing the educational, research,
and clinical activities of the division. It did not feel so much like
extra work, as it added pleasant variety to my daily activities. Adding
to my job satisfaction was developing an even closer connection to
Skinner and Belsey and having a good friend from the Chicago residency join the Thoracic Surgery Division.

This scenario was ideal but was perturbed two years later when
Skinner unexpectedly departed to assume the position of CEO of
New York Hospital. This new role as leader of a major academic
medical center was an important responsibility for him but regretted
by some, including me. It greatly diminished his presence in the
surgical community and, we in Chicago felt, prematurely ended his
tenure as Chairman. He had a successful run developing the department, and becoming a national force within surgery, but might have
achieved even more with the leverage that comes from longevity.
However, a political contretemps with our University's President

over the design of a newly constructed hospital made distant pastures seem greener. There are all too frequently no clear winners in the crunch of academic politics.

The departure of my professional mentor, combined with life-style compromises for my family living through Chicago's winters, weakened the ties to the University sufficiently that I started to look around for my own opportunities to lead a department. I began to interview for various positions, one of which was Chair of Surgery at the University of Nevada School of Medicine. I returned from my first visit pleasantly surprised. The School was relatively young, which implied there were likely to be fewer ingrained patterns, and greater acceptance of new approaches. Subsequent trips confirmed that Las Vegas in 1988 was quite livable and offered a reasonable community life outside of the ubiquitous casinos, so I accepted the position. Having grown up in southern Georgia, near a swamp, dry heat without bugs was quite tolerable.

I began my new job strengthened by having watched Skinner navigate the shoals of academic surgery. From the beginning, I experienced genuine pleasures and rewards. In addition to relishing my continuing thoracic surgical practice, satisfying activities included recruiting quality academic surgeons to the department, and starting new programs such as the first kidney transplant program in Nevada. This was particularly gratifying to me: in 1988, kidney transplants were routine in most of the country but were not being performed in Nevada. Thanks to our new program, patients were no longer forced to travel outside the state to obtain them. By chance (I would have planned it if I could), the first Las Vegas kidney transplant—a success—was on Christmas morning; a good sign for the future of the program. It let the community know we were there: the story was the lead for the Vegas newspapers.

Faculty recruitment is high priority for a medical school in a growth and development phase, as was the University of Nevada. I invested a considerable amount of my time in the process. There were disappointments, as when a sought-after surgeon declined our opportunity, but these were more than made up for by successful recruitments—and the pleasure of getting to know a number of young surgeons starting their academic careers.

Being responsible for the general surgery residency program, especially in the absence of a thoracic surgery residency, led to a close working relationship with these young trainees, and the opportunity to get to know them as people and friends, not just as surgeons. Watching them develop their surgical skills during the five years of the residency reminded me of my experiences. Early on, the faculty and I taught them such basics as tying square knots; by their fifth and final year they had technical proficiency and I enjoyed seeing them master new operations. Most intended to enter private practice, many in smaller communities, so they were after a broad experience rather than focusing on a narrower subspecialty. As time passed and new surgeons swelled the department, I navigated the accreditation hurdles set up by the entities with oversight responsibilities to increase the numbers of residents in our program. Enlarging residency programs is more difficult today. Residents' salaries are paid by Medicare, and a law enacted in the 1990s has capped the number of residents it will support in existing programs of all specialties. This is problematic as physician shortages in nearly all specialties, including surgery, are predicted to be upon us sooner rather than later.

Those were some of the positive aspects of chairmanship. On the less positive side, my major disappointment, or at least challenge, was a struggle with two different groups. One was unanticipated: it was composed of the leaders of the parent university of the medical school. Although the major clinical campus of the school was in Las Vegas, one of the fastest growing metropolitan areas in the country, the parent university was the University of Nevada, Reno. UNR gave the southern campus grudging attention; over time, the school was minimally supportive, hoping to keep the focus in Reno rather than Las Vegas. This was shortsighted; a major opportunity was being neglected. UNR's reaction may have been predictable: for its entire history and until the late 1980s, Reno was the larger of the two cities, and historically the epicenter of politics and development in the state. The remarkable growth of Las Vegas had caught the administration in Reno by surprise.

The more predictable challenge I faced as chair was dealing with private practice surgeons in Las Vegas. These surgeons saw growth of the medical school's department of surgery—with its recruitment of new surgeons—as competing for their patients and their income. All surgeons want busy practices but the reaction in Las Vegas was particularly frustrating and ironic as the explosive rate of population growth in southern Nevada engendered a need and the capacity for more physicians of all types.

This reaction from the private sector was encountered by most young medical school clinical programs during the previous century as they grew, matured, and established themselves in their hospitals and their community. The irony in our case was that our "competition" was in the uncommon situation of a rapidly growing city with plenty of opportunities for everyone. Community memories fade over time and it gets forgotten but most academic medical centers survived this "town-gown" issue at some point in their developmental history.

Although my administrative, teaching, and recruiting duties kept me occupied, I was able to continue a thoracic surgical practice. This was important for several reasons, not the least of which was the sheer enjoyment of operating. This declaration may shock; a nervous patient wants a "serious" surgeon. Don't confuse "enjoyment" with frivolity. My colleagues and I take the responsibility of operating on a human being seriously, but most times we relish what we do. As I anticipated as a medical student, I found genuine pleasure in the acts of dissecting tissues and, for example, completing the removal of a cancerous lung. Interacting with students and residents in the operating room was always gratifying and stimulating and added to the pleasure. More prosaically, having a clinical practice generated additional income (distributed among me, the department, and the school) and kept my "boots on the ground." A chair who is not clinically active quickly loses touch with local hospital personnel, and both local and national practice issues affecting the faculty and residents. An inactive chair will inevitably lose their respect, without which it is impossible to be an effective leader.

In Nevada, I was especially involved with patients with cancer of the esophagus. My interest in this disease had begun during my residency in Chicago. I was drawn to the challenge as a result of my participation in the care of Skinner's many patients. This translated into my own steady involvement with the disease and its surgical treatment when I was in training. However, when I joined the Chicago faculty, it was challenging to compete with my senior colleagues for referrals so my practice there was less than robust. In Nevada, I treated esophageal cancer patients more frequently. Like the chairmanship, this was a mixed blessing: surgical treatment is complicated and technically challenging. I'll go into more detail about my encounters, the evolving biological nature of this devastating cancer, and the surgical interventions for it in my chapter focused on this disease.

There are only a few esophageal diseases other than cancer, GERD, and achalasia. I occasionally dealt with one of these uncommon conditions that is limited to the elderly—Zenker's diverticulum. This is an outpouching of the mucosa that arises between the pharynx (back of the throat) and the upper sphincter of the esophagus in the neck (for those who prefer anatomic to eponymic designations, it is a pharyngoesophageal diverticulum). In appearance, it's as though the mucosal lining was blown out to form a balloon that lies adjacent to the spine, hugging the back of the esophagus.

The diverticulum was first described by Ludlow in 1769, but Zenker got his name attached in 1878 when he elaborated on the condition. This outpouching is the result of pressure building up as aging muscles in the pharynx that control swallowing get out of sync; the upper esophageal sphincter fails to relax in a timely fashion. The pressure increase pushes out the mucosal "balloon." Swallowed food either bounces off a non-relaxed sphincter or gets diverted into the pouch rather than heading down the esophagus. Those afflicted experience difficulty in swallowing. In addition, both food failing to enter the esophagus and pouch contents spilling back into the pharynx irritate the vocal cords, which induces coughing; or are even aspirated into the lungs, resulting in pneumonia.

My representative patient was an 83-year-old lady who was rail-thin after extreme weight loss as a result of difficulty swallowing, had a chronic cough, and had been hospitalized several times for pneumonia. I met her in the hospital after the diverticulum had been found by an x-ray taken while she drank barium. She was disheartened after suffering for years and was eager for the operation I described to her and performed the next day. For this operation,

I made an incision in her neck and dissected toward the spine, where I identified her esophagus and the diverticulum. I excised the diverticulum and cut the upper esophageal sphincter (the muscle of the esophagus where it joins the pharynx)—to limit the pressure the sphincter could generate in the future; one diverticulum was enough. She had to wait a few days to allow some healing but then was able to swallow and eat normally for the first time in several years. I saw her in my office six weeks later; she had gained back most of the weight she had lost and could eat without coughing. Recently an alternative to this operation has gotten some traction. It involves going through the mouth and cutting the tissue between the pouch and the esophagus; I've used this surgical option a few times and found it to be less effective than the open operation.

I relished being a surgeon and chairman. Life in the academic community blossomed as well. I began to get more involved with national thoracic surgery societies and serving on their committees. In particular, I became active in those that included physicians from other specialties and dealt with Medicare to determine the value of operations cardiac and general thoracic surgeons perform. Like sausage-making, you don't want details. Preparing for and participating in the meetings took time—it's a complicated process—but was worthwhile, as Medicare payments are the basis of all insurance payments. Also, it was an opportunity to come to mingle with and know a variety of physicians from other specialties. My job in Nevada was my primary focus but the activity on the national stage was important for my colleagues and a welcome change of pace for me.

12

LUNG SURGERY

In my account of the evolution of chest surgery, I touched on operations for infections in the chest. These interventions were more frequently for infections in the pleural space than in the lung. Early surgeons aimed to drain the infected material, not remove all or part of the lung. This chapter takes us into true lung surgery, its origins and development.

In 1499, seven years after Columbus arrived in the New World, a hesitant Italian named Rolandus described doing lung surgery on an injured man:

> "Called to a citizen of Bologna on the sixth day after his wound, I found a portion of the lung issued [sticking out] between two ribs; the afflux of the spirits and humors had determined such a swelling of the part that it was not possible to reduce it [by returning it into the chest]. The compression exercised by the ribs, retained its nutriment from it, and it was so mortified that worms had developed in it. They had brought together the most skillful chirurgeons of Bologna, who, judging the death of the patient to be inevitable, had abandoned him. But I, yielding to his prayers, and to those of his parents and his friends, and having obtained the leave of the Bishop, the master, and

the man himself, I yielded to the solicitation of about 30 of my pupils, and made an incision through the skin ... Then with a cutting instrument I removed all the portion of the lung, level with my incision."

An unidentified contemporary physician took exception with Rolandus, and expressed a startling therapeutic alternative, feeling he would have:

"... dilated the wound with a small piece of wood, keeping the lung warm with a cock or fowl split down the back ... and kept the wound open till the portion of the lung was wholly mortified."

Except for the unorthodox use of barnyard fowl, this latter approach is actually consistent with the modern standard practice for infected wounds: allow healing by keeping them open until all necrotic (dead or dying) tissue and infected material has spontaneously drained out. This principle applies to the treatment of abscess cavities. What is interesting in this anecdotal report is how experience with accidents like that of Rolandus's patient opened the door to the understanding that elective—not just emergency—lung operations were possible. Although most traumatic events of the magnitude Rolandus's patient experienced must have been fatal, sporadic similar reports appear from as early as his, and continue over the following centuries.

His report and subsequent encounters with similar trauma victims delivered messages important for the development of chest surgery. One was that removal of at least some amount of lung was technically possible; it could be done. The other was that, although one would not expect the survivors of these injuries to be particularly spry, they survived. Early surgeons must have noted there was enough redundancy of total lung function to sustain life—meaning that a person could lose some of their breathing capacity yet expect a reasonable level of activity.

At the same time as Americans were taking up arms for our internecine conflict, an operation by the French surgeon Péan in

1861 was a major advance toward the goal of planned lung resections. His patient had a tumor of the muscle of the chest wall. To Péan's surprise, in the operating room he found the tumor was doing what cancers have become notorious for: growing beyond the muscle, invading and thus firmly attached to the underlying lung. Péan's strategy was to remove the tumor, the involved muscle and ribs of the chest wall altogether (this is called an "en-bloc resection" by surgeons), and, seeking to remove a margin of normal tissue to ensure the whole tumor was excised, he included the lung invaded by the cancer.

Aware they were dealing with a cancer, modern surgeons would anticipate Péan's finding. Cancer is from the Latin for "crab," called that because the natural growth of the tumor into neighboring structures takes place in a way that looks like the irregular outline of a crab. A few years later Block, a Polish surgeon who was probably unaware of Péan's experience, further advanced lung surgery when he successfully removed entire lungs from several rabbits. A major technical challenge was dealing with the lung hilum which harbors three structures: the artery supplying blood to the lung, the vein returning blood to the heart, and the bronchus, the "breathing tube" to the lung. His technique was to pass and tie a stout cord circumferentially around the entire lung hilum, compressing arteries, veins, and the bronchus together, then cut out the lung. His reports and demonstrations of his technique to curious surgeons created a modest stir in Europe but Block's stardom was short-lived. He was persuaded (probably not by as large a contingent as Rolandus required) to operate on his cousin for tuberculosis. We can imagine the enthusiasm with which he attempted to cure a relative. However, as observed by Meade, "unfortunately, his cousin was not as hearty as the rabbits and died." Block was so devastated by the experience, his understandable guilt perhaps exacerbated by the postmortem inability to find any signs of tuberculosis in his cousin, that he committed suicide, prematurely ending what might have been even greater contributions.

Other European surgeons took Block's lead, trying lung resections in a variety of animals—but didn't venture to operate on patients. For example, the Italian surgeon Domenico Biondi operated on 63 animals, including dogs, rabbits, guinea pigs, cats, birds, and sheep. To replicate a common human scenario, he even inoculated some with tuberculosis prior to his operation. Strangely, after demonstrating his ability to perform a successful pneumonectomy in these animals, Biondi never translated his expertise to human patients. Perhaps he was familiar with the unfortunate Block. The occasional chest operations performed on humans were either for infection, trauma or, like Péan, while excising a chest wall tumor to also remove some modest amount of lung invaded by the tumor and thereby attached to it. The real advances were taking place by surgeons working on animals, exploring techniques to eventually be deployed in humans.

What were the challenges to making human lung surgery a realistic achievement? Three technical considerations were the most perplexing and important. We have two lungs; each is composed of smaller units, called "lobes," which are made up of segments. Those are the anatomic landmarks. A question was whether removal of the entire lung (pneumonectomy) was the only possibility—or was it also possible to do something less invasive and take advantage of the anatomical possibilities and only remove a lobe (lobectomy)? Pneumonectomy is actually an easier operation for the surgeon than lobectomy because the anatomic structures that need to be isolated, *ligated* (tied off), and divided are found in the hilum, not buried in lung tissue as is the case for the lobes. During a lobectomy, the search for the blood vessels and bronchus requires teasing apart more tissues; this increases the risk of injuring these structures. Yet removing a whole lung deprives the patient of more pulmonary function than does a lobectomy. This exposes the patient to the risk of pulmonary insufficiency and compromises their life in later years, if activities are limited by severe shortness of breath brought on by even slight exertion. The surgeon (and the patient) would like to preserve as much lung and respiratory function as possible while not compromising the required components of an adequate cancer operation; it was necessary to make lobectomy a safe operation.

The second technical surgical challenge, whether performing pneumonectomy or lobectomy, was how to deal with individual arteries, veins, and bronchi. Should these structures be dissected free from surrounding tissue and be ligated or sutured individually, or was it better to control them by tying a ligature around the entire hilum for a pneumonectomy? The surgeon's control must be perfect during the operation: if not, blood vessels will bleed, and the airway will leak air with each breath.

The anatomic representations in Appendix Two show a lung stripped of its normal overlying and connecting tissues. This is a far cry from what the surgeon encounters. While the vessels and bronchus are more easily found in the hilum than further out in the lung, even in the hilum both the vessels and the airway are sheathed in an envelope of fat, lymph nodes, and connective tissue which shields them from view and binds them to each other. Dissection and separation of the overlying tissues to expose them can result in tears and subsequent, possibly uncontrollable, bleeding. Careful surgical maneuvering through this tissue envelope is required to identify each one, circumferentially clean it of overlying supportive and connective tissue, and then surround each one with a suture.

This also takes time. Time is a luxury afforded by endotracheal anesthesia and the ability we have now to ventilate the lung, which early surgeons of course, did not have. However, the effort is worth it as controlling each artery and vein individually is safer and more secure than a single tie around the whole hilum, which is more likely to slip or fail to adequately compress each vessel. I remember the first few times I was led as a resident through the process of this dissection, always aware an injury to a blood vessel could result in serious bleeding. If I was anxious and tentative with a world-class thoracic surgeon at my side, imagine doing it with no previous experience, no surgical assistant, no anesthetic, and no blood transfusion capability if the worst happened. No wonder the first technique employed was the mass ligature of the hilum. Pneumectomy, despite the drawback of removing more lung, was obviously the better choice long ago!

The final consideration was one that early surgeons understood better following animal experiences: how to close the bronchus so that it was airtight after cutting across it to remove the lung or a lobe. Figure 7 is a cross-section of a bronchus. Note the curved portion of the bronchus supported by rings of cartilage, forming an arch. The ends of the cartilage rings in this horseshoe configuration are

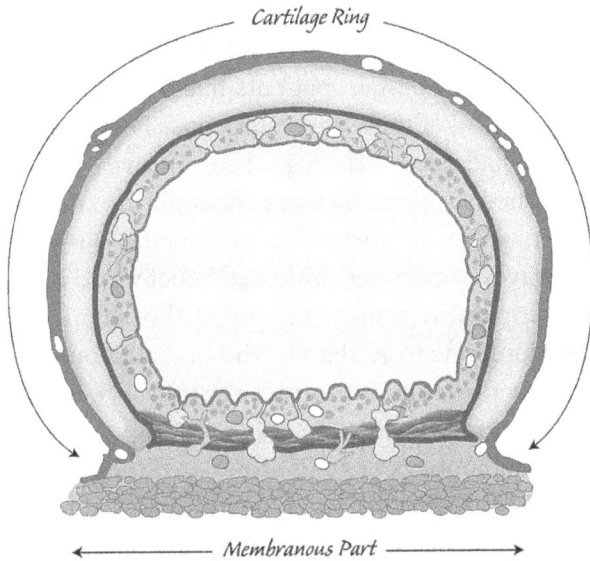

Cartilage Ring

Membranous Part

FIGURE 7.

connected by a flat posterior floor called the "membranous part;" this is a pliable sheet of tissue without any bones or cartilage to make it rigid. The rings are flexible but have enough firmness that they are not fully compressible; they must keep the airways open throughout the breathing process as the pressure inside the chest fluctuates during breathing. Because they are not easily collapsed, tying a surrounding ligature might not reliably close them off entirely. This membranous part is composed of somewhat elastic and malleable tissue which easily conforms to fit the configuration of the underside of the arch of the cartilage rings. The most efficacious strategy is for the surgeon to suture (or staple, in today's world) the membranous part of the bronchus to the inner aspect of the cartilaginous part to obtain a secure and airtight coaptation.

Early operations on animals were important, even essential, steps in the development of the basic techniques for later use in human thoracic operations. There was, however, a dark side to these activities. The surgical community convinced itself that animals felt no pain. It's hard to accept this stated belief at face value, but that was what surgeons espoused for many years. This left surgeons feeling at liberty to lash them down and cut them open without the least attempt to obtain a state of general anesthesia or provide any pain relief. At least human patients had a choice. Or perhaps I shouldn't be so critical of these early surgeons. They were embedded in a society that had such little regard for animals that, for entertainment, it relished such spectacles as cockfighting and bearbaiting. Even worse, surgeons performed experimental surgery without anesthesia on slaves. Again, the professed belief was that these black slaves didn't feel pain. A prime example of this shameful behavior was James Marion Sims in Alabama who operated on many female slaves to develop a procedure to correct a fistula between the urinary bladder and the vagina.

I wonder what motives or goals stimulated these early surgeons to pursue the ability to perform lung operations. Just to take Biondi as an example, operating on and providing care for 63 animals is not a trivial undertaking; it requires time and effort. To know his operations were successful and could be considered for humans, Biondi had to be sure his "patients" survived for the long-term, not just the procedure. He, or someone, had to feed and water the animals, check their incisions, and monitor their recovery.

Surgeons exploring uncharted waters in the hopes of curing a known human disease are easy to understand; there is a need and they have a goal. However, there was no obvious need for a lung cancer operation in the era of Columbus as lung cancer was essentially unknown to the medical profession. Even an 1896 textbook by Paget contains only a passing mention of lung cancer, and no suggestion that surgical intervention would be useful or possible. In 1918, Osler's prestigious medical textbook devoted exactly one paragraph to what is today one of the most common cancers we encounter. Perhaps lung cancers actually were more common, but went undetected, as there was no x-ray capability to discover them. Certainly, no one contemplated operating for them. As we have observed, some chest operations were being performed for various types of infection, but these procedures were primarily to drain out infected material, and only rarely to remove lung tissue. Neither fame, except perhaps fleeting notice in the local medical community, nor fortune would have seemed to reward the surgeon who spent hours mastering lung resection in animals. Instead, I imagine the motive was what drives all pioneer spirits: the irresistible human urge to push the envelope, explore the unknown, and define possibilities and limits. In less noble-sounding terms, they were curious to learn what was possible. While these early surgeons' activities were of little practical use when first performed, their initial forays added to our knowledge base, and they accumulated surgical experience. The result was that established, if rudimentary, techniques were available "on the shelf" when surgeons needed to perform these operations in humans.

In addition to establishing specific techniques, these operations established important surgical principles. One was the value of precision. Ligating or tying individual blood vessels, rather than surrounding and compressing a tissue mass, and placing sutures in an anastomosis in exactly the proper location produce the best possible outcome. Perfection is not attainable. But, for example, when sewing two organs together or closing a cut bronchus, a surgeon is more likely to achieve the desired healing together of the tissues if sutures are precisely the correct distance apart: too close to an edge, they may pull through; too far, and the edges may crumple up and not come together—and tied with the proper tension: too tight, and slicing through tissues is a risk; too loose, and tissues are not brought into sufficient contact. Nature can compensate for minor deviations from the ideal, but patients do better when the surgeon is as compulsively exact as possible.

Surgeons did continue to perform chest surgery for infections, drawing closer to genuine lung operations. Surgery is not an intuitively first choice to deal with chest infections but in the pre-antibiotic era, the only therapeutic options were to drain an abscess cavity or to excise an infected area of the lung. In 1885, another Italian surgeon performed perhaps the first successful lobectomy in a young woman with a tubercular cavity in her right upper lobe. Ironically, she died on post-operative day nine with the diagnosis of carbolic acid poisoning. This diagnosis may reflect the surgeon's attempt to deflect blame away from himself, but it is a legitimate possibility: it was common surgical practice at the time to bathe the surgical field and all exposed tissues with this disinfectant. Perhaps the liquid was considered to be some sort of semi-magical ointment, as the germ theory was far from well understood, or perhaps the folk wisdom, "if a little is good, then more is better," was applied.

The pace of development quickened as the century drew to a close. In 1891, the famous French surgeon Tuffier resected part of a patient's lung for TB by tightening a chain around the middle of the right upper lobe like a lasso. This was not a resection along anatomic lines—not a lobectomy or pneumonectomy—but it was a step closer.

In 1895, the previously mentioned Scots surgeon Macewen operated on a seemingly moribund patient with long-standing TB, and found a lung so riddled with both TB and a concomitant bacterial infection that he was more or less able to scoop out the entire lung with his hands. (Given the amount of infection which must have been present, the blood vessels and the main stem bronchus would have been buried in an inflammatory mass. This would have made it impossible to identify, much less attempt to control, the individual hilar structures. In addition, the pulmonary blood vessels were undoubtedly full of clots so they would not bleed.) The patient went on to survive a complicated postoperative course and eventually recover. While this was arguably not a true surgical pneumonectomy, as neither tissue dissection nor ligation of vessels was performed, the entire lung was extracted. This again demonstrated the ability for a patient to survive and function after such a profound loss of respiratory capacity. Emboldened, surgeons performed a small number of similar procedures in which diseased and end-stage lungs or lobes were essentially scraped out.

Macewen made many contributions to surgery, perhaps most importantly to the fields of neurosurgery and orthopedics. (No one specialized in a single type of surgery in those early days.) As a student of Lister, he was an early, strong proponent of surgical antisepsis and definitely an early leader of thoracic surgery. He was also a man not to be taken lightly outside the operating room. As related by Harley Williams, Macewen was once in a railway carriage with two ladies and a loudly offensive drunk. After persuasion failed to calm the offender, "he placed his two thumbs inside the mouth of the drunken fool and dislocated the man's lower jaw so that he sat absolutely dumbfounded and silent with his mouth compulsorily open for the rest of the journey. Then by an equally skilled surgical manoeuver, the jaw was liberated." Yikes!

One of his most influential acts, as far as American surgery is concerned, is something Macewen did *not* do. He was offered the opportunity to be the first professor of surgery at the newly opened Johns Hopkins Medical School and Hospital—but he declined. If he had accepted, the world would probably only know William Halsted, Hopkins's second choice for the position, as the drug addict who squandered his surgical potential. Halsted famously became addicted to cocaine while experimenting on himself to determine its potency as a local anesthetic. Yet despite his inability to shake his addiction, Halsted was enormously influential. As Chair of Surgery, Halsted developed a resident training paradigm that changed how surgical residents learned their craft, at Hopkins and across our country, since Hopkins was then, as it is now, a medical institution frequently emulated by others.

As per Halsted, no longer would a poorly defined and unstructured "apprenticeship" be sufficient. Training would henceforth take place in University hospitals with defined faculty, and include a process of supervision, instruction, and progressive responsibility. Halsted also introduced seminal, innovative surgical techniques (for hernia repair and breast cancer, among others) and emphasized the importance of handling the patient's tissues with care and gentleness, a tenet now called "respecting the tissues." Halsted's residency system was extraordinarily competitive and arduous. A beginning class of interns was pared down as the years passed until only one remained. He—always he—lived in the hospital and was available continuously until Halsted deemed him ready to move on, typically to head his own department. (A reminder of the origin of "resident.") The whole process of becoming a surgeon took a decade or longer. Halsted's training philosophy remains influential today but "pyramidal" structures for residencies have been superseded by what are called "rectangular" programs: all first-year residents have the opportunity to complete the program.

Perhaps inspired by Macewen's success, in 1908, a British surgeon performed a thoracotomy on a young lady with fulminant infection of her lower lobe of the left lung. The cause was blockage of the bronchus, by a tooth she aspirated during a dental extraction, which allowed bacteria to proliferate in the obstructed lung. The surgeon applied four clamps to control the blood vessels and the bronchus to the infected lobe and the lobe was excised. Rather than suture the chest closed, the thoracotomy was left open with the clamps protruding between the ribs. On postoperative day three, the clamps were removed without adverse consequences (such as bleeding from the cut ends of the blood vessels), and the patient continued to recover. Clamping blood vessels, rather than ligating them, with delayed removal of the clamps, was a surprisingly common and usually successful surgical practice of the time, though it defies common sense. Presumably enough tenacious blood clot formed in the clamped blood vessels to block the open end.

Despite the encouraging early days, the patient died of infection on the 28th day after the operation. The type of infection was an empyema, an infection of the pleural space, inside the chest but outside the lung. Although not recognized at the time, one explanation for the postoperative infection is the lack of continual drainage of the pleural space. This is now routinely obtained following a lobectomy by placing an argyle chest tube into the thoracic cavity through a small incision separate from the thoracotomy. Its free end is connected to a suction device to enhance its effectiveness in draining the pleural space. In addition to providing immediate evidence if untoward bleeding should occur inside the closed chest, the tube provides two additional benefits. It drains out air escaping the lung so that accumulating air cannot compress the remaining lung. And, importantly, the tube keeps the lung fully inflated and evacuates infected material so that a serious infection cannot brew inside the chest.

The lung lobes are not separate entities like slices of bread in a loaf. There are tissue bridges between them which must be cut across to remove a lobe and some postoperative air leakage from those sites is inevitable. Air accumulating in the chest but outside the lung is called a "pneumothorax." As air accumulates it builds up pressure and becomes a tension pneumothorax which compresses the remaining lung to the point of collapse so it cannot function properly. Increasing pressure can even shift the mediastinum away from the operated side, distorting the two major veins returning blood to the heart so that they kink and close off just like your hose when watering the lawn. Without blood returning to it, the heart has no blood to pump out to the body, and the patient goes into shock. The chest tube fills an essential role by removing this air, keeping the lung inflated, and giving the raw lung surface time to heal—which stops the air leak. For both prevention of infection and pneumothorax, the chest tube provides a vital service that was only recognized in later years.

Separating them from other tissues and ligating the pulmonary artery and vein separately proved to be safe and a more secure technique for controlling blood vessels than mass ligature of the entire hilum. For closing the bronchus, sewing the malleable posterior membrane to the firm, cartilage-supported part was identified as the most reliable technique and the least likely to allow air to leak out. In 1912, Morriston Davies in England utilized these techniques of individual ligation of blood vessels and suturing of the bronchus as he performed a right lower lobectomy for a lung cancer which had been found by the recently introduced x-ray machine. This would have been the first successful operation for lung cancer had the patient not developed the seemingly inevitable empyema and succumbed on day eight. Encouragingly for future efforts, postmortem examination showed the artery, vein, and bronchus were closed and in an appropriate stage of healing. The techniques worked. Two years later, a survey of the world's surgical literature determined that 16 operations, either lobectomies or non-anatomic lung resections, for bronchiectasis (the once more common, localized, pneumonia identified in Chapter Seven) had been reported with half the patients surviving. Going forward, anecdotal reports of these procedures were forthcoming. By the early 1920s use of a chest tube, with its salutary benefits, was becoming a routine addition to lobectomy operations.

In 1923, Evarts Graham, a leader of American surgery of whom we shall learn more, reviewed the world experience and found 48 reports of lung resection for bronchiectasis with "complete success" in only eight (17%) patients, with a 52% mortality rate. Again, half the patients didn't survive the operation. Not encouraging. The following quotation in the same year from the President of the American

Association for Thoracic Surgery describing the typical experience provides insight into why these operations for bronchiectasis were so fraught with poor results.

> "The patient is placed on the operating table. There may be cyanosis. It induces coughing. The anesthetist is greeted by an evacuation of a large amount of pungent, purulent sputum, incident to the posture on the table. The whole bronchial tree may be filled with this material as the anesthetist begins [and] … the pleura is no sooner opened and traction on the diaphragm commenced, than the need of general anesthesia is obvious. As the secretions well toward the trachea, the cyanosis increases. The lower lobe obstinately resists being delivered; the pleural adhesions are strong and widespread; the attachments to the diaphragm are ropelike and tenacious. Finger dissection is inadequate. Work with the knife and scissors is blind. Cleavages are sought in vain. The pericardium is dangerously involved in the adhesions.
>
> "Meanwhile, the patient's condition may become distressing and perhaps alarming. If open pneumothorax is adding insult to injury, the lung cannot be used to plug the thoracic gap, because the lobe is not deliverable.… The mucopurulent secretion may interfere with the respiration under positive pressure. And then the difficulties multiply.… There is bleeding and infectious leakage from the lung, and bleeding from the diaphragm. Tight closure of the chest without drainage seems inadvisable under such conditions, and yet necessary to avoid the ills of postoperative pneumothorax. Suddenly, it is obviously time to return the patient to his bed. Not much has been accomplished."

This daunting scenario was clearly intended to discourage the dilettante surgeon—certainly, it would dampen my enthusiasm. The message was that lung surgery was an undertaking for only real men (still no women surgeons around). Perhaps, as a result, reports of lobectomy continued to appear only sporadically. By the late 1920s, these experiences did at least, however, finally nail down the benefits and absolute need of inserting a chest tube following lobectomy.

Ultimately, in 1931, the same Rudolf Nissen who helped advance surgery for benign esophageal disorders reported the first successful true pneumonectomy. His patient was a 12-year-old girl with chronic bronchiectasis who actually suffered a cardiac arrest during an initial attempt at removing her lung. She was resuscitated and underwent the successful operation two weeks later when Nissen ligated the hilum and supplemented this with silk ligatures. Surprisingly, he left the lung in place. Deprived of its blood supply, the lung died and spontaneously sloughed off several weeks later. Resilience in both patient and surgeon was a requirement for this accomplishment. One year later, Haight at the University of Michigan duplicated Nissen's feat using an identical technique. It again required two operations to get the job done, as the first attempt was aborted when the patient's pulse rate shot up to 168 beats/minute. Clearly these operations stressed these two patients to their maximum limits, both of whom must have been severely debilitated by their chronic infections. I also imagine the two surgeons were more than a little stressed themselves. But they persisted and thoracic surgeons were prepared to deal with lung cancer.

13

Lung Cancer

The thoracic surgical wave crested when Evarts Graham took the stage. This leader of American surgery became the Chairman of Surgery at Washington University in large part because of his renown as the head of the Empyema Commission for the Army during World War I. This chest infection—empyema—was a frequently lethal complication of battlefield thoracic injuries. The Commission established treatment principles emphasizing closed chest tube drainage (with the end of the tube outside the patient placed under water, not left open to the air) rather than a major open thoracotomy to drain the pus. Both military and civilian surgeons adopted this recommendation with the result that the morbidity of this condition was greatly reduced.

In 1933, at Barnes Hospital in St. Louis, Graham performed the first pneumonectomy for lung cancer (and the first one-stage pneumonectomy) in a 49-year-old obstetrician. A primary lung cancer at the origin of the left upper lobe bronchus had been confirmed by looking into the airways with a bronchoscope. Graham didn't have today's flexible instrument which is easy to direct out several generations of bronchi. He had to rely on a rigid tubular bronchoscope but was able to find the cancer in the left lung where the main stem bronchus split into upper and lower lobe branches. This new procedure added to the surgical armamentarium the important capability, combined with x-rays, to be more certain of the exact location of a lung tumor. The patient was realistic about his situation; in preparation for his operation, unbeknownst to his surgeon, he purchased a burial plot. However, he must also have been reasonably confident as he proceeded despite being advised by Graham's resident the night prior to sign out of the hospital because of the likelihood of not surviving the procedure. Using endotracheal anesthesia, Graham performed a left thoracotomy. Once in the chest, he felt the tumor mass where he expected, where the bronchus to the left lung split to supply the upper and lower lobes. To extract all the cancer, he had no choice but to remove the entire lung. He applied two clamps across the hilum of the lung, thus controlling the pulmonary artery, the two pulmonary veins, and the bronchus. After cutting between the clamps, the left lung was removed through the open chest. There must have been a moment of silent awe as those at the operating table viewed for the first time in history the spectacle of an empty chest in a living person. (I can't imagine this happening in Macewen's operation, as his patient's chest was collapsed and constricted by all the inflammation.)

Graham's operative note describes his placing, perhaps after a deep breath or two, three "transfixing" sutures around the hilum and through the bronchus, removing the clamp and placing radon seeds to treat any residual cancer left behind. A few ribs were removed to allow some collapse of the soft tissues of the chest wall to decrease the amount of empty space left behind. The patient's postoperative course had only a few bumps. An abscess in the chest cavity was drained two weeks later and more ribs were removed 10 days after that to collapse the chest wall even further. Finally, after just over two months in the hospital, the patient—sustained by his remaining right lung—walked out in good condition and resumed his medical practice. The final pathological examination of the removed lung confirmed the lung cancer and also found that it had spread to nearby lymph nodes. Despite the diminished prognosis caused by the presence of lymphatic spread, the patient's cancer never recurred; in fact, he eventually outlived his surgeon. Although Graham had established the feasibility of this operation, the bloom soon came off. His next several patients were consecutive fatalities, which led to the sobriquet of the Butcher of Barnes Hospital. If the first patient had also failed to survive, lung resections would surely have been put on hold.

Graham is an important figure in the history of American surgery for other clinical achievements than the pneumonectomy. There are two of particular note. He was the co-developer of the first radiologic method to image the gallbladder, using a radio-opaque material which was taken by mouth and concentrated in the gall-bladder so that it would show up on an x-ray. This technique made it possible to diagnose acute cholecystitis (inflammation or even infection of the gallbladder). This test was eventually superseded by the use of ultrasound, but it was an enormous advance at the time. Additionally, working with a medical student (whose idea it was), an epidemiologic study of his lung cancer patients was one of the first to establish a correlation between smoking and lung cancer. The proof of actual causation took more time than necessary. The first obstacle to overcome was the vigorous suppression of evidence by the tobacco companies. Secondly, in the early limbo between correlation and causation, it was actually thought plausible that lung cancer led to smoking. The theory was that the tumor irritated and caused inflammation of the airways; this was the cause of the coughing and could be soothed by smoking. Graham's seminal work substantiated the belief in this etiologic connection held by his colleague Alton Ochsner, another prominent surgeon of the day, who, perhaps apocryphally, is reputed to have said that "the only excuse for smoking is being on fire."

During his chairmanship at Washington University in St. Louis, Graham defined the mission of medical school faculty by championing the importance of their commitment to research. He advocated what was called the full-time system: faculty surgeons were fully or partially supported by the medical school, freeing them from the necessity of generating income from patient care, providing time for teaching and research. Like Halsted at Hopkins, he advocated transitioning resident training from an unstructured, preceptorial process to an organized multiyear training program with progressive and graded responsibility. He was involved with, and even participated in the founding of, several medical and surgical societies, national councils, and committees, and served as a consultant to governmental bodies. However, despite this body of work, he is relatively underacknowledged no doubt because, although respected, he was intensely disliked by many. The reasons for this are not a mystery. Descriptions of his behavior reveal him as frequently condescending and arrogant, willing to harshly criticize perceived flaws in others and unable to tolerate opposition or disagreement. Graham was a smoker all his life; the ultimate irony occurred when a nagging cough was determined to be the result of lung cancer, which ended his life in 1957.

One final observation: In 1940, Graham, like Macewen before him, was offered but declined the position of Chair of Surgery at Hopkins. In this case, chairmanship landed in the hands of Alfred Blalock. This likewise greatly affected the course of surgical events as, at Hopkins, Blalock merged his surgical skills with the physiological insights and encouragement of the pediatrician Helen Taussig to develop the first operation for blue babies. If he had remained where he was (at Vanderbilt, in Tennessee), this serendipitous interaction would not have taken place, the Blalock-Taussig shunt would never have been developed, and the first operation for blue babies would have certainly been delayed.

As the surgical community became aware of Graham's milestone achievement, other surgeons were encouraged to follow suit; they began to perform successful operations for lung cancer. It was a good thing that this precedent of lung resections had been established as they seemed to be suddenly needed. Either the incidence of lung cancer increased exponentially or, as the availability of chest x-rays to find lurking tumors proliferated, detection improved. Probably both. The seeming explosion of lung cancer was due in large part to the inexorable growth of the tobacco industry and the increasingly widespread acceptance of cigarettes. Despite the industry's aggressive attempts to conceal and deny the relationship between smoking and lung cancer, it has become clear that between 80% and 90% of lung cancers are caused by exposure of smokers or bystanders to the *carcinogens* in the smoke. Although not the most common cancer, lung cancer is so lethal that it kills more people in the USA than any other malignancy.

How does this heinous smoke do what it does? Cigarette smoke contains more than 5,000 (yes, that's the correct number of zeroes) different chemicals. Is it surprising to learn that more than 70 of these are carcinogenic? They exert their effect primarily by damaging the DNA inside the cells of the airways, allowing them to replicate without restraint. Particularly bad actors are the chemicals benzene and the nitrosamines. For good measure, certain other chemicals in the smoke such as arsenic and nickel interfere with the cells' ability to repair injured DNA. Smoke is more like a shotgun than a rifle: if one component doesn't get you, another will. And the total impact of cigarette smoke isn't limited to the smoker: just being in the neighborhood of a smoker is dangerous, as passive exposure also increases lung cancer risk. To twist a popular expression, it's all bad. Surgeons and medical oncologists work to develop cures but that is only possible for a minority of patients; prevention is the ideal.

Thoracic surgeons, learning from operations in animals, realized that lobectomy was technically possible. Surgeons had learned it was safe to dissect and control the individual blood vessels and bronchus to each lobe—a practice preferable to Graham's mass ligation of the hilum. As surgeons gained experience with both pneumonectomy and lobectomy, lobectomy was established as the preferable operation for cancer. We have upper, middle, and lower lobes in the right lung, but only upper and lower lobes on the left. In a lobectomy, the lobe removed is identified by the side of the body it's on, and its upper, middle, or lower location, in a description such as "a right upper lobectomy." Rather than having to sacrifice an entire lung, extracting only a lobe and allowing the patient to retain the other lobe(s) of the lung maximized the patient's postoperative breathing capacity and quality of life. Importantly, experience showed that lobectomy did not compromise the likelihood of curing the cancer as long as all the malignancy was removed.

In fact, Belsey, who reasoned his way to his Mark IV operation for GERD, used his uncommon surgical skills and knowledge of anatomy in 1939 to co-develop a method for an anatomic lung resection even smaller than a lobectomy called a "segmentectomy." (As you might expect, this means the removal of one of the segments of a lobe.) This operation is ideal for treatment of bronchiectasis where no margin of normal tissue around a cancer is required. Thoracic surgeons, however, occasionally perform segmentectomy for lung cancer when it is thought (or hoped) to be adequate for cancer removal, and the patient doesn't have sufficient lung capacity to tolerate a lobectomy, much less a pneumonectomy. There is a trade-off as the cure rate is somewhat less than for lobectomy, perhaps because fewer lymph nodes can be removed. Also, residual cancer in the remaining lobe may be left behind.

In 1950, Belsey also showed that it was possible to excise portions of the trachea and the two main stem bronchi to each lung for cancer. He removed substantial lengths of both trachea and bronchus in patients to remove cancers localized within them. He replaced the missing tubular airway segments with an innovative reconstructive technique. He implanted tubes he constructed from wire coils between the two open ends of the airway which were too far apart to be sutured back together. He then wrapped the wire coils with *fascia* from the leg. All his patients survived; their lives were extended. To my knowledge, this was a feat of surgical legerdemain never repeated by another surgeon even though Belsey's accomplishment was seventy years ago.

Lobectomy is established as the ideal operation for lung cancer for most patients. It gives the best chance for control of the cancer while sacrificing the least amount of lung to get that result. But there is a need for surgical flexibility. There are instances when alternative surgical options are more appropriate. A patient with marginal lung function may be left with insufficient breathing capacity if an entire lobe is removed, much less an entire lung. In that case a segmentectomy (or what is called a "wedge resection," in which a pie-shaped wedge of lung around the tumor is removed) becomes the surgeon's choice.

On the other hand, there are times only a pneumonectomy will suffice for the thoracic surgeon to accomplish a complete resection, leaving no malignant cells behind—an essential requirement if an operation has a chance of curing the cancer. Segments of bronchus or even trachea can be removed but of course this means sewing together the open ends of the remaining airways to preserve their continuity—unless you're Belsey. As mentioned, lung cancer can penetrate the lung lining, the visceral pleura, and invade an adjacent structure. If the cancer growth is into an organ that the patient can't live without, like the heart, then an operation is rarely wise. If the invaded structure is the rib cage then complete removal of the cancer is still possible, but the surgeon must remove the ribs and muscle, leaving them attached to the lung, at the same time the lobectomy is performed. This is the opposite scenario from Péan's experience where a tumor of the chest muscle was invading the lung.

Thoracic surgeons can do all these operations. When should you use them? Before recommending surgery for a patient some questions need to be answered. Is a cure obtainable? Is the patient fit enough to come through a lung resection? Should the patient receive chemotherapy or radiation treatments before surgery? An operation for lung cancer should only be performed if the patient is fit enough to survive it (and expect a reasonable quality of life afterward) and the cancer has not spread beyond reasonable resection limits so that there is an expectation of cure. The fitness of patients is evaluated by multiple examinations, and they are put through a battery of tests particularly focusing on the status of the heart and the breathing effectiveness of the lungs; two organs weakened by years of smoking which we see in nearly all patients. If this evaluation determines that the patient's condition is sufficient to safely undergo an operation, the next consideration is the likelihood of a cure; there is no value to an operation if it does not provide a chance for a complete eradication. Removing all the cancer does provide this possibility. This is most likely to be the case when the tumor is contained within the lung (not growing into a structure outside the lung such as the rib cage) and has not spread through the bloodstream to other organs or through the lymphatic system to lymph nodes in the mediastinum. If any malignant cells are left in a patient after an operation, the cancer will inevitably recur, and the patient will not have benefited from the operation.

The process of defining the extent to which the cancer has or has not spread, developing the road map the surgeon uses to determine the likelihood that all cancer can be surgically removed, is called "staging" the cancer (this has nothing to do with the theater). There are typically two aspects to the staging process. The first is searching for evidence of spread through the bloodstream in the form of distant metastases in other organs, most frequently the liver, a bone, or the brain. Metastases can be suggested by patients' symptoms, such as a new headache implying a metastasis in the brain and detected with increasingly sophisticated radiologic examinations such as computerized tomographic scans (CT), magnetic resonance imaging (MRI), and positron emission scans (PET), in addition to chest x-rays.

Metastases define Stage IV and signal that surgery would be futile. Removing the primary tumor would not help the patient: even if only a single metastasis is large enough to be identified by the scans, and it also could be removed, there are always more that are too small to show up on the scans and will inexorably proliferate. Truly solitary metastases are rare.

Chemotherapy or radiation therapy are the standard treatment for patients with metastatic disease. Rarely curative, these modalities can prolong life. New options being investigated include drugs which interfere with the cellular metabolism of cancer cells, and different forms of immunotherapy which harness the body's own defense systems. DNA analysis (genotyping) of the tumor cells to determine their susceptibility to these therapeutic options is increasingly and helpfully used to personalize a patient's treatment.

The second aspect of staging after looking for spread to other organs is to evaluate the lymph nodes around the lung, especially those in the mediastinum. The status of these lymph nodes is determined from the same PET, CT, and MRI scans, direct biopsy of the nodes, and a sampling of them with a needle passed through an airway during a bronchoscopy. When there is involvement of the lymph nodes adjacent to the lung or in the mediastinum but there are no metastases to other organs, we call this an intermediate scenario or stage (Stage II or III). This is because it is between the two extremes of a cancer in the lung with no spread (Stage I) and one with distant metastases (Stage IV).

The body's lymphatic system normally transports excess fluid and waste products of metabolism from the tissues back to the blood vascular system. Cancers shed malignant cells which are picked up by the lymphatic system to be swept away like a leaf in a stream. The lymph nodes along the way filter out particulate matter including these cells and are loaded with immunologic weapons which can attack—hopefully to eliminate—bacteria and cancer cells. Experience has shown that surgery alone is rarely curative for lung cancer patients in the presence of spread to nodes in the mediastinum, even without distant metastases. Perhaps a third of patients who present with an initial diagnosis of lung cancer are in this category. An operation alone will not cure these patients.

However, rather than abandon all hope of cure, these intermediate-stage patients are candidates for what is described as a multimodality approach. They are treated initially with a either radiation therapy or chemotherapy or both together. Surgery is then considered if the patient is fit enough, and the neoadjuvant therapy has killed enough of the cancer that it is possible for the surgeon to remove all residual cancer in the lung and lymph nodes. Results to date suggest this aggressive approach is beneficial, especially for those patients who respond to the preoperative treatment with impressive regression of the cancer. It is an arduous experience for the patients, who must endure the side effects of radiation and chemotherapy only to undergo a major surgical procedure. If restaging (repeating the battery of investigations) shows that the tumor or lymph nodes failed to respond to the initial therapies or the patient is not fit enough for this strenuous program, then surgery is withheld, and the treatment is continued chemotherapy and/or immunotherapy, the efficacy of which continues to improve.

Only about a quarter of patients with newly diagnosed lung cancer have Stage I disease and between 35% and 40% are in Stage IV with the remainder mainly in Stage III. To dramatically increase the number of patients we cure, we need therapies that can eradicate metastatic disease. To get this we must have a greater understanding of the process of metastasizing.

When and why cancers spread (metastasize) are subjects of intense investigation. The answers could lead to interventions for prevention or treatment. We know cells frequently escape from most cancers, including lung and esophageal cancer, resulting in the dissemination of malignant cells into the bloodstream on a regular basis. However, a cancer can be present for variable lengths of time, sometimes even years, before a metastasis forms in a distant organ. One may never develop. Is the reason for this erratic behavior because only some of these circulating cells have the potential to survive unattached to the primary tumor? Or is the key, alternatively, that they must find themselves in an organ capable of providing the right environment to nurture them to settle in and thrive? After all, metastases are more likely to be found in some organs, such as the liver, than in others such as the kidney.

As the problem is frequently posed, is the difference the seed or the soil? Is a metastasis due to a property of a circulating cancer cell, or determined by where the cell takes root? If we understood this biological process, it might be possible either to prevent metastases from developing or eradicate them once they have been detected. We do know that as a lung cancer enlarges, it is more likely to metastasize—but small ones can metastasize, and large ones not. Unlocking this mystery would be a major step forward in our ability to care for, even perhaps cure, more lung and esophageal cancer patients.

How effective is thoracic surgery in curing lung cancer? This question is most meaningfully considered taking into consideration the stage of the cancer. When the patient's cancer is Stage I the tumor is within the lung (not invading into a neighboring structure), there has been no spread to lymph nodes, and no metastases are present. Approximately 70% to 80% of patients can expect to be alive with no evidence of cancer five years after their operation. Results worsen as the stage advances. The least successful operations are for Stage III patients who have spread of the cancer to lymph nodes. (Remember, patients found in Stage IV have metastases and are not surgical candidates.) Only about a third of these patients are even candidates for surgery, and the five-year survival in this group receiving an operation as part of the triple modality program is less than 50%. This is the big picture; these are the "facts." As an experience of mine illustrates, for patients it's about more than facts and statistics.

I knocked and walked into the exam room. For me, literally another day at the office. Not so for the occupants. My new patient LC is perched in one chair, hands clenched in her lap, and her husband sits fidgeting on another. We all knew why we were there: LC had lung cancer. She is 72 years old and has smoked for most of them. I had reviewed all her radiologic scans obtained by the referring oncologist—easy to do nowadays, on an office computer; the days of searching for x-rays in the radiology suite are over.

Her scans showed a tumor in the right upper lobe of the lung with no evidence of metastases to other organs or the mediastinal lymph nodes. Assessments of her heart and lung function showed both to be working well enough for her to be able to come through a lobectomy with a reasonable quality of life. As we talked, her body began to unclench but her husband remained on edge. I explained the planned lobectomy: its need, the risks, and the hope and probability—but not certainty— of a cure. We scheduled the procedure.

In the operating room about a week later, with the patient on her left side, I performed a right thoracotomy, slicing through her skin and muscles before spreading apart the ribs. The tumor was immediately visible. Using a special breathing tube, the anesthesiologist allowed the right lung to collapse as he ventilated only the left lung, giving us more room to operate. The surgical resident and I cut into the connective tissue of the hilum of the lung until we found the main artery and two veins going to the right lung. We dissected into the fissure separating the lobes, cutting through connective tissues, until we could identify the arterial and venous branches to the upper lobe, pass silk sutures around them, ligate (tie the sutures), and cut them. After stapling and dividing the bronchus, we removed the lobe. We removed collections of lymph nodes from the mediastinum, but none appeared abnormal. I was surprised to note almost two hours had passed; I was lost in the moment.

I spoke reassuringly to LC's husband in the waiting room but reminded him she wasn't out of the woods. On the second day after her operation, the patient became short of breath, lightheaded, and her blood pressure dropped. Evaluation showed her heart rhythm had changed from a normal pattern to an irregular one called "atrial fibrillation," compromising her heart function. Her husband was caught by surprise; patients' families fixate on the risk during an operation when in fact, it is extremely unusual for a patient not to survive the operation. The surgeon is most anxious during the first few days afterward, for that is when complications occur. Disruption of heart rhythm occurs in a small number of lobectomy patients for uncertain reasons. Medication given over several hours converted her heart back to a normal rhythm and the remainder of her hospitalization was uneventful. The pathologic exam of the lobe and removed lymph nodes classified the patient as having Stage I squamous cell carcinoma of the lung.

LC was a typical patient, and she did well even though her hospital course included the heart event. The majority, but not all, patients have a similar experience. Despite fear and anxiety, their operation is uneventful, and a few days later they go home. LC was representative for another reason. When I saw her in my office six months after her operation, I could smell cigarette smoke: she had resumed smoking despite vigorous warnings about the risk of a new lung cancer. When challenged, she admitted her addiction was too strong and she couldn't resist despite our warnings and her husband's concern. This frustrating scenario is all too common and speaks to the continuing frequency of lung cancer deaths.

Minimally invasive surgical techniques, as discussed in Chapter Seven, are superseding open thoracotomies such as the one I performed. Patients have much less pain—less cutting, no rib-spreading— after a chest operation, go home sooner, and return to normal life activities quicker. Nothing is lost, as the likelihood of obtaining a cancer cure is unaffected. Chests won't be "cracked" as often in the future, as residents trained in operating this way move into and populate the general thoracic surgery field.

Treatment of lung cancer continues to improve. Although eradication of smoking and the lung cancer it causes would have the maximum impact on survival, early detection of tumors greatly benefits patients. Low-dose CT scans (which minimize radiation exposure) in smokers older than 55 years can find lung cancers in an earlier stage than those not detected until symptoms develop. Cancers in less advanced stages are more likely to be cured. More and more efficacious chemotherapeutic drugs are available. Immunotherapy is becoming an effective addition to the armamentarium. Minimally invasive operations provide excellent outcomes for patients with limited disease.

Yet any discussion of lung cancer should end by re-emphasizing that prevention is far better than treatment and at least 80% of lung cancers are caused by cigarette smoke. While individuals have the right to choose to put themselves at risk, smoking is a public health problem. Not only is the smoke harmful to bystanders, there is a considerable cost to society: the obvious is the financial cost of the cancer treatment. In addition, there is the loss of productivity as the patient leaves the workforce, not to mention the unnecessary loss of life. All this must be taken into consideration by society and balanced against the personal freedom to choose to smoke.

On a more personal note, it was painful as a thoracic surgeon to share the pain felt by patients and their families as they dealt with a death sentence, when they might otherwise have enjoyed more happy years together if cigarettes had not been part of their lives.

14
▾

ESOPHAGEAL CANCER

April, as per T.S. Eliot, may be the cruelest month—but there is no doubt cancer of the esophagus is the cruelest cancer. Its impact is brutal. To start, it's a killer. If not treated, it is quickly lethal. In the 1980s, when I finished my residency, the overall survival rate five years from the time of diagnosis was less than five percent; that's a 95% death rate. Things haven't improved much.

There's more. It's a particularly cruel malignancy as, in addition to its lethality, it tortures the unfortunate patient. Although relatively uncommon, esophageal cancer causes extreme suffering, and significantly impairs quality of life during the short time the patient struggles for survival. As these cancers grow inside the esophageal *lumen* and progressively obstruct the passageway, the patient's symptoms inexorably progress from a painful difficulty swallowing solids to complete obstruction to everything the patient tries to get down. Not only is the sufferer weakened by not getting adequate nutrition but is eventually dehydrated from even being unable to swallow liquids. Without treatment, patients simultaneously starve, and suffer the indignity of choking on their own saliva. Early operations removing part or all of the lung were not invented to deal with cancer. Rather, over time, surgeons applied them to lung cancer. In contrast, surgeries removing any part of the esophagus, all termed an esophagectomy, *were* developed specifically to deal with esophageal cancer.

Esophageal cancer has plagued humans for millennia. Over 2,000 years ago it was identified in China where, Hurt notes, it was said, "Those discovered ... in the autumn will not live through the next summer." In the West, Galen in the second century described "fleshy growths" which obstructed the esophagus. While this malignancy was known, no treatment, surgical or otherwise, was possible or even contemplated. Beginning in the late nineteenth century the noted Austrian surgeon Theodor Billroth, a surgical giant, was the first to attempt esophageal resection. He began by performing resection of short segments of the *cervical* esophagus in the necks of dogs. He chose to operate in the neck to avoid the problems associated with entering the chest, particularly the inability of the dog to breathe with an open chest. His experience bore fruit when one of his former assistants, a man named Czerny, became the first surgeon to successfully apply to a patient the lessons they had learned from these operations on dogs.

In Germany in 1877, Czerny excised from the neck of a human patient a segment of the cervical esophagus containing a cancer. The proximal, open end of the esophagus was sutured to the skin—an esophag*ostomy*—so that the patient's saliva and everything she swallowed drained out into a bag. The patient survived a year feeding herself by pouring liquids through a rubber tube surgically implanted into her stomach. A first therapeutic step had been taken but it did not constitute much of a surgical triumph as it must have been an unpleasant year for the patient. The woman's life was prolonged, but its quality was surely dismal. The search for a way to reestablish continuity, reconstructing, or replacing the missing portion of the esophagus, was a major challenge for thoracic surgeons who began to master the technique of esophageal resection—esophagectomy. As elaborated below, this is a problem unique to extirpative surgery of the esophagus (that is, an operation for the purpose of removal, whereas in operations for GERD or achalasia, nothing is removed). Elsewhere in the gastrointestinal tract, for example in the small intestine, when the surgeon removes a segment, the two ends of the mobile and redundant intestine are easily brought together and rejoined by suturing or stapling them together to restore continuity. It's not so simple to do this in the esophagus.

Continuing to focus their efforts on the esophagus in the neck, Billroth and his trainees performed a small number of cervical resections—with no patient surviving longer than a year. In 1886, another of Billroth's pupils, von Mikulicz in Poland, removed a length of esophagus in the neck for cancer and then closed the gap he had created with a tube fashioned from the patient's skin which was left connected to its blood supply so that it would survive. This was a complex undertaking; it did allow the patient to swallow and eat for the few months he survived. Perhaps emboldened, 10 years later, Mikulicz turned his attention to a patient with a cancer of the esophagus in the chest. He removed the lower esophagus and its junction with the stomach—the cardia—and sutured the remaining esophagus to the stomach. However, following the operation the patient quickly succumbed to peritonitis, infection in the abdominal cavity, probably caused by leakage of saliva and gastric juices from the anastomosis.

As in the early days of lung resection, these disappointing results discouraged the surgical community sufficiently that only sporadic reports of attempts at esophagectomy followed. All were neck operations, and the high mortality rate persisted. Most patients who survived the operation struggled mightily as there was no reconstruction of the missing esophagus to provide the ability to eat so nutrition arrived through tubes. A few were provided with the complicated skin tubes that restore continuity of sorts. A report in 1898 noted only 10 esophagectomies for cancer had been reported. Even if a few had been missed or gone unreported, it is clear that progress was only incremental and tentative.

In 1902, two surgeons in France resected cancers of the thoracic esophagus from their respective patients. Both forays into the chest were equally unsuccessful: there were no attempts at reconstruction, and both patients expired within 24 hours. These operations failed but the French surgeons had taken on the important challenge for thoracic surgeons: how to accomplish resections of the esophagus in the chest. Most of the esophagus, and therefore most esophageal cancers, are in the chest. The capability to successfully carry out intrathoracic esophagectomies was necessary to make a difference for the majority of patients.

Sauerbruch, the man who devised the negative pressure operating chamber, in 1905 removed segments of the thoracic esophagus in a series of operations in dogs. He showed that the two open ends could not simply be sewn together because the excess tension caused by stretching them across the surgically created gap resulted in the sutures pulling through the tissues of the esophagus. When this *dehiscence* occurred in a patient, leaking saliva would cause a life-threatening infection. This difficulty does not arise when two ends of the small or large intestine require connection. The intestines can easily be mobilized by cutting them away from their tissue attachments, and the two open ends put end to end and sutured together without any tension pulling them apart. There is no such possibility in the esophagus because it is fixed in place and has no redundancy: removal of a segment creates an unbridgeable gap, and thus a surgical challenge.

Sauerbruch creatively solved the tension question by using the stomach as a replacement. Rather than attempting to stretch the ends of the esophagus together, he advanced the stomach, after separation from its attachments below the diaphragm, upward through the esophageal hiatus and anastomosed it to the transected esophagus. This maneuver was to eliminate the tension which follows an esophagus-to-esophagus anastomosis, and thereby diminish the likelihood of a dehiscence and resulting infection. Although he made this procedure work in dogs, he was never able to translate his success to humans; the three patients on whom he operated did not survive. However, his groundwork pointed the way forward to solving the reconstruction challenge.

Evidence that Sauerbruch was on the right track was strengthened that same year, when a Chicago surgeon, operating in dogs and on cadavers, described successful use of the stomach for reconstruction.

He did not use the entire stomach but trimmed away part of it so that the gastric remnant resembled a tube. This was a helpful contribution to the goal of removing all possible cancer as this action also removed the lymph nodes that are in that location. The tube was closer to the configuration of the esophagus it was replacing; we now know it functions better in this shape as patients swallow better than when surgeons use the entire stomach to take the place of the esophagus. However, no one picked up on this information. By 1910, in addition to ongoing dog trials (evidence of continuing interest), a surgical review noted a paltry total of only 21 reported esophagectomies for cancer, performed either without reconstruction of the alimentary tract or with the aforementioned skin tubes, just 11 more than those reported 12 years earlier.

In 1913, barely more than a century ago, Frans Torek, a surgeon in New York, through a left-sided thoracotomy excised a cancer of the esophagus in the chest. The patient survived; this was a game-changer. Torek had established that the extirpative aspect of the chest operation was feasible. After removing the segment with the cancer, he was left with the esophagus coming down from the mouth, the esophagus going down to join the stomach, and a gap in between. Picture cutting out the midsection of a hose: one part would be connected to a faucet and the other no longer attached. He simply sewed closed the opening in the esophagus leading to the stomach. It would not be needed to function any longer. He then performed what surgeons call an exteriorization of the esophagus coming from above (the proximal end). This means he brought it through the muscle of the anterior chest wall and sewed the opening or mouth of this proximal esophagus to the skin; anything swallowed would drain out through the esophagostomy.

One pervasive shibboleth had been put to rest. The vagus nerves (from the same Anglo-French word that gave us "vagrant") originate in the brain, one on each side, pass through the neck and chest and end in the abdomen. These wandering nerves affect multiple organs in their course, one of which is the heart; when stimulated they cause it to slow. Both adhere closely to the thoracic esophagus; the surgeon operating on the esophagus in the chest would by necessity manipulate them. A widely held concern was that unavoidable vagal stimulation would cause the heart to stop and be immediately fatal. As Torek stated in the report of his operation, "The dreaded vagal collapse had ... been safely avoided." What relief there must have been in the operating room! To provide fluids and nutrition during postoperative recovery, the patient received the standard (for the times) course of enemas consisting of a mixture of hot coffee, strychnine, and whiskey.

The colon does not absorb; its job is to store and evacuate. This means the attempt to provide nutritional support was ineffective. On the other hand, the inability to absorb this bizarre cocktail containing the poisonous neurotoxin strychnine—thought at the time to be in the right dose a stimulant much like coffee (though you won't find it offered by your local barista)—prevented it from slaying the patient. More effectively, fluids were also administered through a gastrostomy tube in the stomach. The patient survived all this and lived another 13 years, although with a limited lifestyle.

Torek's patient is shown during recovery from surgery in Figure 8. Her appearance is distressing; it demonstrates the extreme state of emaciation typical in patients with esophageal cancer if treatment is delayed. Of note is the external tube connecting the cervical esophagostomy to the gastric tube. Food swallowed by the patient exited the esophagus and descended this tube to arrive at the stomach. This was the patient's sole means of obtaining nutrition for the remainder of her life. It's as if Rube Goldberg had been put in charge of the reconstruction. Nonetheless, as it is set forth in Ecclesiastes, "A living dog is better than a dead lion," and the patient survived over a decade using this apparatus. By 1948, a total of 58 "Torek esophagectomies" had been performed—with a daunting mortality rate of 71%. Three-quarters of patients never left the hospital after surgery. Clearly, this would never be the final answer.

An ingenious alternative approach to Torek's was described in 1933 by the British surgeon Grey Turner. (He gets credit although, apparently unknown to him, there was a similar report earlier in the German medical literature.) Turner based his approach on thoughtful consideration of the anatomy of the mediastinum and the esophagus and relied on his surgical experience to guide him. Rather than entering the chest through a thoracotomy, he worked from the

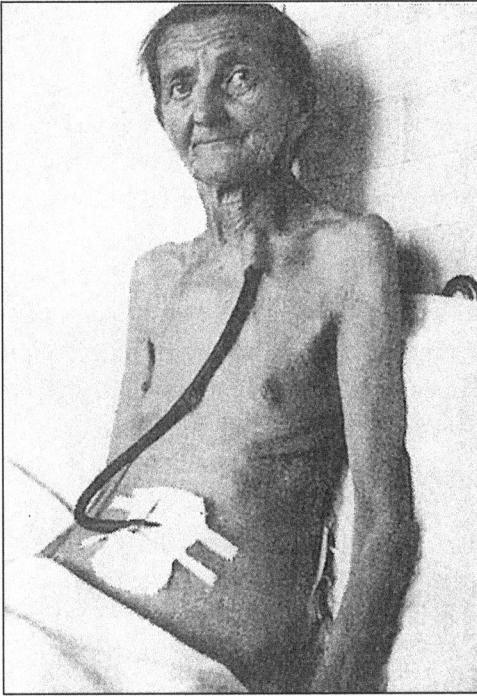

FIGURE 8.

two ends of the esophagus. He approached the cervical esophagus through a neck incision and the abdominal part of the esophagus through an abdominal incision (a laparotomy). The esophagus was detached from tissues down from the neck and up from the abdomen through the esophageal hiatus. To attack the out-of-sight mid-portion, he inserted his hand through the hiatus in the diaphragm, behind the heart and into the mediastinum. His hand having disappeared from view, his experienced fingers carefully teased the esophagus free from its tissue attachments in the mediastinum.

Considering that the esophagus is contiguous with the aorta, the pericardium around the heart, the trachea, and several large blood vessels, Turner's approach required perfect knowledge of anatomy, a hand sensitive enough to know how much force the tissues could tolerate before catastrophe, and more than a little bravery. Any injury to the neighboring organs was irreparable as the operative field was inaccessible, fully shielded by the sternum. His words capture the moment:

"... finally, it was necessary to introduce the whole hand into the posterior mediastinum and to practice the manoeuvers of the obstetrician separating a retained placenta, before it [the esophagus] was eventually loosened and could be withdrawn into the abdomen where it hung loose.... Its withdrawal was followed by a gush of blood but this soon stopped.... [This] disclosed an enormous yawning cavern, in and out of which air rushed with a terrifying and disconcerting noise."

Grey Turner reconstructed the esophageal defect by creating a skin tube that ran from the esophagostomy in the neck, down the front of the sternum, linking up to the stomach in the abdomen. Not many of these types of esophagectomies were performed by Turner (or anyone else) for a long while. Interest in his technique was revived in the 1970s and was regularly employed by some surgeons. It is now known as the transhiatal esophagectomy. The dissection and removal components of the procedure used today are the same as those described for the original experience. Grey Turner's skin tube technique has been discarded, however, and for reconstruction the stomach is pulled up to the neck through the now empty route of the esophagus, through the posterior mediastinum, and anastomosed to the stump of the cervical esophagus.

I consider this feat by Grey Turner astounding for the originality required to think of it (his experience with using his hand to extract retained placentas from the uterus after childbirth clearly played a role), the audacity required to attempt it, and the skill necessary to bring it off. Now there are textbooks describing the technique, and experienced surgeons to guide the learner. These were uncharted waters for Grey, and there were lions and tigers lurking.

Here is what I mean: when Grey's hand entered the mediastinum, it was immediately squeezed between the heart above, the spine below, and the aorta to the side. Any blunt finger pushed into the tissue tethered to these structures could tear them with the possibility of immediate major hemorrhage, or a fatal tear in the trachea. Audacious behavior, therefore to do so, yes, but backed up with skill and preparation. One would expect Turner to have been a forceful and dominant personality but his obituary paints a different picture: a soft-spoken, "short man who dressed shabbily and wore an ancient bowler on the back of his head. He used to cover his teacup with his bowler hat to keep the tea warm!"

A surgical milestone was passed in the late 1930s when the first two successful resections of the esophagus in the chest with simultaneous reconstruction were carried out. The techniques used by the surgeons were similar in both operations. Marshall, in 1937 in Boston, was first to accomplish this feat but Phemister at the University of Chicago frequently gets the credit as he presented his 1938 operation at a society meeting and published an article about it in the leading thoracic surgery journal before Marshall described his own success. (It's not often that Boston surgeons are beaten in the publications race for precedence. For example, the Massachusetts General Hospital experience with ether anesthesia discussed in Chapter Six was published the subsequent month.) Both surgeons operated through the left chest, dissected the esophagus free from its attachments to neighboring tissues, and resected a length containing the cancer. The stomach was then reached through an incision in the diaphragm. As with the esophagus, the surgeons separated the stomach from the surrounding tissues (which required dividing several of its blood vessels while leaving enough to maintain viability). Each surgeon then pulled the now-untethered stomach up through the hiatus into the chest, where it was anastomosed without any tension to the free end of the esophagus. This esophagogastrostomy (the joining of the esophagus to the stomach) healed, both patients survived and were subsequently able to eat and swallow in a normal manner: a more enjoyable life than being encumbered by external tubes.

Less than a decade later, in 1946, the British surgeon Ivor Lewis introduced a logical and significant technical advance. Because the aorta, as it leaves the heart, curves from the right to the left side of the chest before proceeding down into the abdomen, it crosses the esophagus in the mid-chest and blocks the surgeon's ability to get to it from the patient's left side. This limitation precludes operating on carcinoma of the middle esophagus using a left thoracotomy. (Both Marshall's and Phemister's patients' cancers were low down near the esophagogastric junction, and a left thoracotomy provided sufficient exposure of the operative field.)

For his operation on a patient with a tumor halfway down the esophagus, Lewis began with a laparotomy, ideal for preparing the stomach for subsequent transposition into the chest. The laparotomy was then sutured closed, the patient rolled on his side, and Lewis performed a right-sided thoracotomy. Going through the right chest provided Lewis a view of the entire length of the esophagus without the aorta in the way. With unimpeded access he was able to transect the esophagus high up in the right chest. It is of value to divide the esophagus in a location which maximizes the distance from the cancer. The longer this cancer margin (the length of the esophagus from the cancer to where the esophagus is cut across), the greater is the likelihood that all malignant cells have been removed. Lewis grasped the previously prepared stomach through the hiatus and pulled it up into the right chest where he joined it to the esophagus (an esophagogastrostomy). This Ivor Lewis operation has stood the test of time. The combination of an abdominal beginning to prepare the stomach, excising the lymph nodes near it, with a right chest approach to dissect the esophagus and remove thoracic lymph nodes is by far the most frequently employed method for esophagectomy for cancer worldwide.

A modification of the Ivor Lewis procedure, the McKeown procedure, is to add a third, cervical, incision so that the gastric interposition can be anastomosed to the esophagus in the neck. Experience with the two techniques has identified a conundrum that remains unsettled. When an esophagogastrostomy does not heal properly, the resultant leak of swallowed saliva and gastric juice can result in overwhelming infection, sepsis, and death. Not surprising as the human mouth contains a variety of virulent bacteria. (One of the first lessons a surgeon learns in emergency rooms is that, while a dog bite can safely be cleaned and sutured closed, closure of a human bite often results in an infection because of its bacterial load.)

Experience suggests that anastomotic leaks are less common from anastomoses in the chest than in the neck; however, when they occur they are more likely to have devastating consequences. There are several reasons. First, leaks into the small neck space form an abscess which is quickly identified as the patient's temperature rises and the wound reddens and becomes tender. The surgeon acts on this early manifestation to start treatment early, before the infection can spread. The signs of a leak into the chest are more subtle and can take longer to identify, which delays intervention. Second, chest leaks contaminate and infect a significant amount of tissue in the chest and mediastinum while leaks in the neck are more contained. Finally, treating a significant chest leak frequently requires a return to the operating room to close the leaking anastomosis. In contrast, opening a neck incision and packing it with gauze—usually at the bedside without a trip to the operating room—provides a generally successful means of evacuating the leaking contents and usually is curative.

When the surgeon describes an operation as an Ivor Lewis or a McKeown type, it identifies where the incisions are placed. No operative details regarding the surgical activities inside the abdomen or chest are indicated. This is not a trivial issue as there are important surgical choices regarding the amount of tissue surrounding the esophagus (especially lymph nodes) to remove. Early operations aimed to remove the cancerous portion of the esophagus blocking food from passing and, eventually, restore normal swallowing with a gastric interposition. Surgeons did not go out of their way to remove the adjacent lymph nodes and other tissue. Pioneer surgeons were pleased simply to have their patients survive the operative challenge and leave the hospital able to swallow. Cure of the cancer was welcome but unexpected. Occasional patients did enjoy a lengthy life, but most succumbed to cancer recurrence within a year or two.

This pessimistic surgical attitude persisted through the 1980s; the sole realistic goal of surgery, associated with a high rate of complications, was considered to be palliation. Rather than to cure, an operation was performed to restore the patient's ability to swallow for their remaining—nearly always short—life. This was a frustratingly incomplete goal but did improve some patient's quality of life, if only for a limited time. Cure was considered a happy instance of good fortune and only achieved in 10 to 20 percent of the operated patients.

An Edinburgh thoracic surgeon named Andrew Logan began to stretch the paradigm with his description in 1963 of an operation designed to go beyond palliation and actually cure the cancer. His operation was extensive with removal of the esophagus with neighboring lymph node groups and tissue such as the diaphragm, pleura, and the surrounding fat and connective tissue complex that can harbor unseen lymph nodes. His approach followed the surgical principle espoused by Halsted for a cancer operation. Halsted recommended removal of tumors with tissue around them—so that there was no chance of failing to remove all cancerous invasion—and regional lymph nodes which could harbor metastatic disease before it spread systemically. In Logan's series of esophagectomies, 51% of operative survivors lived for five years, sufficient time to consider them cured. This was a substantially improved outcome compared to those of his peers. Unfortunately, the other side of the coin was a prohibitively high operative mortality rate of 25%. Fully a quarter of his patients never left the hospital after their operation. This was an unacceptable trade-off. The surgical community paid little heed and his approach lay fallow for a decade. But one surgeon had seen the Holy Grail; none other than my mentor-to-be, David Skinner.

While on the faculty at Johns Hopkins in the 1970s, Skinner began to focus his interests on surgical treatment with the aim of curing esophageal cancer. Having spent time learning from Belsey, and influenced by Logan, he was ready. His operative approach mimicked Logan's strategy of sweeping up surrounding tissue, mainly clumps of lymph nodes, together with the esophagus, but used McKeown's three-incision technique for maximum exposure of the operative field. I learned this aggressive approach from him as a resident and began to employ it when I joined the Chicago faculty. At that time, pessimism permeated the international surgical community: cure was an unexpected bonus following esophagectomy. We, especially Skinner, persevered in Chicago. Early results were acceptable but were not all that was hoped for: mortality for the first 30 days after surgery hovered around 10%, and the five-year survival rate between 20% and 25%. Yet this experience made two important contributions. The goal of cure was now established as part of the conversation. No longer would it only be about palliation; Skinner had permanently shifted the paradigm. The thoracic surgical community noticed.

In addition, the Chicago experience identified important differences in outcomes for patient subgroups. Those with no, or only a few, lymph nodes harboring metastases had better survival, i.e., were more likely to be cured by the more extensive operation, than by other thoracic surgeries using the traditional procedure which left more lymph nodes and other tissue behind. This strongly suggested that there was a benefit to removing adjacent lymph nodes along with the esophagus. This was called a "regional lymphadenectomy."

The modern era had begun but change wasn't overnight. Through the 1980s, for most surgeons, the goal of surgery remained palliation. Cure was still considered a happy instance of good fortune. The actual operation, esophagectomy, was itself a considerable hurdle for patients to get over. These lengthy and technically difficult operations challenged both surgeons and patients as suggested by Earlam's 1980 meta-analysis: "Oesophageal resection for squamous cell carcinoma has the highest operative mortality of any routinely performed surgical procedure today." This was the gloomy background Skinner, and eventually others, had to supplant with strategies leading to potential cures.

As with lung cancer, so with esophageal cancer: an operation is only beneficial if all malignant cells can be removed. An esophagectomy is not going to cure patients with metastatic cancer. Therefore, as with lung cancer, accurate preoperative staging is essential. Even if only a single metastasis is detected this is a result of cancer cells still circulating in the blood and smaller, as yet undetectable, tumor deposits are inevitably growing elsewhere, out of reach of the surgeon. Similarly, a surgical cure is not achievable for those patients whose tumor invades organs adjacent to the esophagus such as the aorta. We can look for this with endoscopes that provide an ultrasound view of surrounding tissues from within the esophagus. Subjecting these patients to a futile operative procedure can only complicate a limited life span with pain and hospitalization. We want to keep these patients out of the hospital and at home with their families.

The status of the patient's regional lymph nodes is also an important factor in determining therapy. Endoscopic ultrasound, using a needle attached to the endoscope to sample suspicious nodes through the wall of the esophagus, allows evaluation of lymph nodes in the vicinity of the tumor. The exact number associated with a diminished prognosis is debated but it is certain that more than five lymph nodes with metastatic cancer is an ominous sign. These patients are equivalent to those with metastatic disease and only eligible for an operation if they have a dramatic response to chemotherapy with or without radiation therapy. Chemotherapy is also usually recommended when the pathologist finds lymph node involvement. As I said at the outset of this chapter, esophageal cancer is an especially harsh challenge for patients. The morbidity and mortality associated with esophagectomy have historically been at the highest end of the thoracic surgical spectrum. There are multiple reasons. Some include factors related to the patient. With both obstructed swallowing limiting the ability to eat, and a malignant process gnawing away, the typical patient is malnourished and lacks nutritional reserve. The operation requires entry into the chest so that both the heart and lungs are stressed. Older patients, especially smokers, do not tolerate this well. Finally, there is an anatomic consideration. The esophagus lacks a serosa, the outside covering present on the remainder of the gastrointestinal tract; it is more tenuous to suture as it lacks this supportive tissue layer. This makes devastating leakage from the anastomosis with the stomach more likely than for other gastrointestinal anastomoses.

The picture looks better now. Thoracic surgeons have improved the procedure. The perioperative mortality rate for esophagectomy has decreased considerably from earlier days and is less than five percent in experienced institutions. There are multiple causes of this improvement. Patients receive more aggressive nutritional support before and after their operation, and we are able to provide better critical care support in the intensive care unit and hospital as they recover. We have accumulated surgical experience, and technique has improved as has technology; surgical staplers used in constructing anastomoses have been an important addition. And the outlook for those coming through the operation has improved. The five-year survival rate of patients undergoing surgery has increased significantly to nearly 50%. Accumulated experience suggests that Logan's and Skinner's belief that survival is enhanced when tissue is removed in which lymph nodes lurk is correct. Accordingly, most surgeons perform a regional lymphadenectomy during the esophagectomy. This improvement in treatment results could not have come at a better time as the incidence of this cancer—the number of new cases—has been on a steady rise.

When the cancer has spread or patients are not fit enough for an operation to be safe, they are not abandoned. Palliation to improve the quality and prolong the life of a patient becomes the goal. Newer and better chemotherapy drugs are being developed; some are already in use. Radiation therapy can shrink the primary tumor and be used to relieve pain when directed against metastases in a bone. Some patients have a complete remission with these therapies, particularly when combined, meaning that no cancer is detectable by the battery of scans and endoscopy. Unfortunately, nearly all these patients relapse; but this effect gives hope for the future. If the patient is unable to swallow because the tumor is completely blocking the esophageal lumen, both chemotherapy and the radiation treatments can shrink the tumor, although this takes some time. As either a permanent or temporary measure, a tubular, expandable metal mesh device called a "stent" can be placed during an endoscopic procedure to hold the tumor open sufficiently to accommodate liquids and soft food while the other therapies are having their effect. This option is preferable to using a tube placed into the stomach through the abdomen. This "G tube" does provide caloric support but requires the patient to live with a protruding tube and denies them the ability to enjoy eating.

Over the last two years, two changes have made it harder to assess the seemingly improved results of esophagectomy. First, new, effective chemotherapy for esophageal carcinoma is now routinely given, frequently in combination with radiation therapy, before an operation. (This neoadjuvant therapy is given to all patients except the rare patient thought not to have any lymph nodes involved.) Esophagectomy is not performed if patients do not respond sufficiently to this regimen. We learn the response by repeating the battery of radiologic and endoscopic exams to look for the persistence of too many involved lymph nodes, nodes outside the operative field or the development of metastases. This so-called" multimodality approach" has been shown to improve the cure rate regardless of the type of operation, especially in patients who respond with significant tumor regression prior to a resection. So, it's not the esophagectomy alone that's responsible for improved results.

The second change is a shift in the biology of esophageal cancer, perhaps reducing its aggressive behavior. Thirty years ago, as I got involved, the majority of esophageal cancers were found in the mid-portion of the esophagus, halfway between mouth and stomach, and arose from its lining, which is a squamous epithelium exactly like skin. At present, esophageal cancers in the USA, and the Western world in general, are much more likely to be found in the lower esophagus near the gastroesophageal junction and arise from the glandular epithelium, such as lines the stomach. This epithelium produces what are termed adenocarcinomas, meaning they are formed by glandular cells. We don't know why this shift has occurred; we do know that it has been coincident with an increase in the detection of what is called Barrett's esophagus.

Norman Barrett, a British surgeon in the middle of the last century, operated on a small number of patients who required esophagectomy for an ulcer in the esophagus. Unexpectedly, he found that the esophageal lining in these patients resembled that of the stomach: the epithelium of their lower esophagus was composed of glandular, rather than squamous, cells. This abnormal epithelium subsequently has been shown to be associated with GERD and to have the potential to degenerate into adenocarcinoma.

Over the past several decades the incidence of Barrett's esophagus has dramatically increased. A current speculation is that the West's epidemic of obesity, a risk factor for GERD, has increased the numbers of patients with acid reflux. Acid reflux can lead to the development of Barrett's esophagus by injuring the normal squamous epithelium, which is replaced by new columnar epithelium with a tendency to become unstable and form cancer. In contrast, in Asia, where obesity is less prevalent, Barrett's esophagus is rarely identified, and most esophageal cancers are still of the squamous variety. In Japan, for example, cancer of the esophagus is one of the most common tumors, and well over 90% are of the squamous type.

What to do when Barrett's esophagus is found in patients? Although there is the potential for malignant transformation, most patients do not actually develop carcinoma. Performing an esophagectomy, with its risks and morbidity, in all patients would be excessive. The current standard is to extensively biopsy the abnormal epithelium at the time of esophagoscopy. (This is a reason that an esophagoscopy with a close examination of the esophageal mucosa should be performed on patients newly diagnosed with GERD.) If cancer is identified, it is treated according to its stage.

If, however, there is no evidence that the epithelium is evolving toward forming a cancer by exhibiting dysplasia—a condition where some cells show early neoplastic changes—then no treatment other than for GERD is indicated, although repeat esophagoscopy is important every few years for surveillance purposes, in case Barrett's dysplasia or early cancer develop. Finally, if dysplasia is present there are several options. The most popular today is endoscopic therapy, not surgical resection. The abnormal cells are either ablated with a laser during endoscopy, or the abnormal esophageal lining is separated from the overlying muscle and removed through an endoscope. Following either of these interventions, the patient is treated either medically or surgically for GERD, and we keep an eye with repeat esophagoscopy over time to detect any return of the Barrett's epithelium or cancer development.

The quality of life for patients after an esophagectomy varies but is typically good or at least reasonable. Most eat a regular and unrestricted diet although they fill up quickly—part of the stomach has been removed so its capacity is diminished; smaller meals are better tolerated than a few larger ones. The stomach not only has less capacity, but it is also now in the chest. As the lower esophageal sphincter is always removed by the operation there is no longer any native anatomic barrier to prevent the stomach's contents from simply spilling up into the mouth. To diminish the likelihood of regurgitation and subsequent aspiration of gastric contents, patients are counseled not to lie down or go to sleep soon after eating so that the stomach has time to empty. Occasionally there are complications related to the operation, the most common of which is scarring of the anastomosis of the esophagus to the stomach, causing a stricture which requires dilation (stretching with a balloon or a tapered rubber device) during an endoscopic procedure. Less frequently, after esophagectomy, due to the unavoidable cutting of the vagus nerves which control gastric emptying, the stomach may fail to function properly so that food isn't passed normally into the small intestine. This can usually be treated with drugs to stimulate the stomach muscles to contract more forcefully.

The encouraging conclusion is that esophageal cancer treatment is both safer, with lower perioperative mortality rates, and more likely to result in a true cure than just a few years ago. We aren't sure whether this gratifying improvement is due to the use of multiple treatment modalities, more aggressive operations which incorporate removal of lymph nodes, a change in the biological nature of the cancer, or a combination of these factors. Probably all three contribute. And the quality of life after esophagectomy is much improved from earlier years.

I have intimated it can be challenging and somewhat stressful to care for and operate on patients with esophageal cancer. The operations are lengthy, taking between five and six hours of intense concentration. In the 1980s, patients were thin to begin with and their cancer nudged them toward emaciation. Most patients nowadays are larger, even obese, so even a significant weight loss leaves them heavy. Fat obscures the anatomy, covering the normal planes between organs, increasing the difficulty of finding and safely controlling blood vessels. And it's not over when they leave the operating room. Surgeons have to be alert to heart and lung complications, much like following lung procedures but more so because of the length of the operations and the effect of operating in both the abdomen and chest. The most worrisome potential complication is a leak from the anastomosis of the esophagus to the stomach. The use of stapling devices to replace sewing them by hand has reduced the frequency of leaks but every time the patient's temperature rises the surgeon is anxious. These observations don't mean I didn't like performing esophagectomies—just that the degree of difficulty intraoperatively, and concern postoperatively, was greater than for most procedures.

My experience with patient EC is illustrative. I first saw this 70-year-old woman in my office. Her progressively difficult and painful swallowing led to an endoscopy by a gastroenterologist who diagnosed an adenocarcinoma in her esophagus, near where it entered the stomach. Metastatic disease was ruled out by scans but endoscopy with a needle biopsy also identified cancer in a nearby lymph node. Under the care of a medical oncologist she was treated with both chemotherapy and radiation. Repeat evaluation in six weeks documented shrinkage of the tumor and the lymph node with still no metastatic spread. Because of the combined effect of the cancer and her treatment, she lost thirty pounds but still weighed two hundred pounds.

I began the operation with her flat on her back. My first incision was from the bottom of her sternum to just below her umbilicus. I had two goals to accomplish inside the abdomen. The first was to sepa-rate the esophagus—the location of the tumor—from the diaphragm at the hiatus, while preserving a layer of normal tissue around the cancer to ensure I left no malignant cells. The other objective was to cut the stomach attachments to the spleen and colon and divide some of its blood vessels so that I could move it into the chest, a process called mobilizing. The biggest challenge was dissecting through EC's fatty tissue to be sure as many lymph nodes as possible remained attached to the stomach and its major blood vessels. I was slightly tense during this phase but, as usual, it was satisfying to tease and cut apart the tissues until the stomach's largest artery and vein were carefully dissected free and cut between two ligatures, again keeping all lymph nodes (which tend to cluster around blood vessels) with the tissue to be removed. The entire undertaking, including making and suturing the incision and inserting a tube in her intestine for admin-istering food as she recovered, took about two hours.

We closed the abdominal incision and repositioned her on her left side. I performed a thoracotomy on her right chest. Ribs were spread apart and the anesthesiologist, using a special tube in the trachea, excluded the right lung from ventilation so it collapsed down, improving my access to the esophagus. I encircled the tubular esophagus with a rubber strip high in the chest, far from the tumor. Working down toward the diaphragm, I cut the attachments of the esophagus, holding it in place, being sure to encompass visible lymph nodes as well as fatty tissue areas known to harbor unseen nodes. Using stapling devices that deliver a quadruple row of staples and cut between the middle two, I divided the esophagus a good distance above the tumor. I pulled the stomach, free of attachments, through the diaphragmatic hiatus and, using the same stapling device, I excised part of it below the tumor. This allowed me to remove most of the esophagus and some of the stomach with the tumor and attached tissue containing lymph nodes and created the gastric tube I described previously. Using other stapling devices, I anastomosed the end of the esophagus to the stomach, placed a chest tube, and closed the thoracotomy. Another two and a half hours.

We extubated the patient (removed the breathing tube from her trachea) in the operating room but she left well connected to the outside world: two IVs, the chest tube, a Foley catheter to drain her bladder, and the tube in her intestine used for feeding. She spent an uneventful night in the intensive care unit, although I was called at 1 a.m. by the resident who reported her urine output was low; we agreed she needed more IV fluids, and that solved the problem. Instilling a nutritional liquid through the tube in her intestines helped maintain her strength in the subsequent postoperative days. She steadily recovered after that, but on the fourth day her temperature shot up. Worried about a leak from her anastomosis, I obtained an X-ray with her drinking barium. The anastomosis was intact; we found her fever was due to an infection of the tip of her IV in a vein. The fever resolved when we removed the IV.

EC went home on the seventh day after surgery and progressed her diet from liquids to soft foods to regular food over the subsequent weeks. Pathological examination of the tissue removed at her operation showed only a few malignant cells where the tumor had been, and a small number in one lymph node. Because of the lymph node involvement, we gave her a short course of adjuvant chemotherapy. All was well for six months, until she began to notice that when she ate, her food stuck on the way down. My evaluation found narrowing at her anastomosis of esophagus to stomach due to a stricture—scar tissue build-up. This was stretched open during an esophagoscopy, and her swallowing returned to normal. At one year, she felt well and there was no evidence of cancer. She ate all foods but was more comfortable with four small meals a day, rather than the standard three.

I am sure, as with other operations, that minimally invasive techniques are steadily replacing open operations such as the one I just described. Minimally invasive esophagectomy is more technically challenging than thoracoscopic lung operations, but it also will undoubtedly become the standard.

15

SWEAT

D on't sweat it. Good advice aimed to turn anxiety down a notch. Contained in this encouragement is the message that sweating reveals excessive concern. Better not to sweat. But this is not good advice if taken literally. In fact, sweating is a salutary process, even if sometimes unpleasant and socially embarrassing. You may not like living with sweat, but you literally can't live without it. Those liquid beads are there for a reason. Our ability to sweat is critical to regulation of our body's temperature. Our body and its organs are built to function within a temperature range: extremes of cold (hypothermia) and heat (hyperthermia) are dangerous and potential lethal. The evaporation of this liquid on the skin is the cooling mechanism that combats overheating and makes life more comfortable in mild heat; in extreme temperatures, it is a life-saving physiological process. If the body temperature rises to excessive levels, internal organs begin to fail and eventually shut down. So sweating is a good thing—but you *can* have too much of a good thing. And that's where thoracic surgery comes in.

As with any bodily function, the sweating process can go awry. Sweat, a mixture of water and salt, is produced by the two to four million sweat glands scattered around our bodies just under the skin. These glands can really put it out; they are capable of secreting two to four quarts per hour and 10 to 14 quarts per day. Sweating is mediated through a component of the nervous system called the sympathetic system, itself part of the autonomic nervous system which works automatically, without conscious effort. The sympathetic nerves to the body arise from a chain of nerves that lies outside of but adjacent to and parallel to the spine. (The spinal cord is inside the bony spine.) The anatomy of the sympathetic chain is shown in Appendix Two.

A nerve chain is much thinner than, but has the appearance of a piece of string with a series of knots at regular intervals. The knots are ganglia (singular: ganglion) which are collections of nerve tissue made up of *neurons*. Neurons are the cells that are the basic unit of the nervous system; they transmit action messages from the brain to the appropriate body part. The string is the extension of the neurons that connect the ganglia to each other. Spinal cord nerves communicate with the sympathetic ganglia through extensions they send out of the spine. The brain sends instructions down the spinal cord and out these extensions to the sympathetic chain. Depending on the brain's assessment of bodily and ambient temperature, the sympathetic chain communicates action messages from the brain to the sweat glands through the network of nerves which emanate from the ganglia and run outward to the body surface. The glands are either stimulated to produce more sweat or are downregulated or even turned off if conditions are right.

How does chest surgery fit in? Thoracic surgeons are occasionally called on to treat hyperhidrosis—the disorder when the body's sweat glands overdo their job and produce sweat when cooling the body is not necessary. It is estimated that hyperhidrosis affects approximately three percent of the population with no known predilection for gender or ethnic group. The 97% of us free from hyperhidrosis experience reasonable amounts of sweating at appropriate times. This keeps us from overheating and even moistens our skin to help keep it soft. Not so for those afflicted with this idiopathic process who are unfortunate enough to be inappropriately drenched in sweat, more in hot climates but even in air-conditioned buildings. The cause has not been identified but is speculated to be an abnormal brain response to emotional stress which gets translated into hyperactivity of the sympathetic nervous system so that the glands, which themselves are normal, are excessively stimulated and sweat comes pouring out.

The vascular system is also caught up in this. Our multitasking sympathetic nervous system plays another role besides regulating sweat gland productivity; it also modifies the size of blood vessels by either constricting or relaxing them. Squeezing them down decreases their cross-sectional diameter; this is essential to maintaining an adequate blood pressure when a person goes into shock from blood loss. If the vessels retained their normal size during blood loss, there would not be enough blood to fill them to capacity, and blood pressure would drop. This ability of the sympathetic nerves means that when they are inappropriately stimulated to rev up sweating in hyperhidrosis, they also constrict the small arteries in the skin in the vicinity of the affected sweat glands. The end result is an area of skin that, in addition to being sweaty, is cooled not only by the sweat evaporation but also by being deprived of the benefit of circulating warm blood which squeezed down vessels have diverted away.

I was aware of this uncommon disease but had not cared for a patient until a young man, who was soon to enter college on a music scholarship, came into my office in Las Vegas in the mid-1990s. It's one thing to read about a disease; meeting a patient puts meaning to the words. As we introduced ourselves, I found myself holding a very distinctive hand which immediately told me his diagnosis. Clammy doesn't suffice; his hand was distinctly cool and, most striking, was more than damp. It was saturated; sweat dripped from his fingertips. As I spoke with him and his mother, they made it clear that this was a significant social handicap, and a cause of embarrassment and emotional anguish. (Picture the scenario holding hands on a date.) In addition to its social and emotional impact, the condition was a major stumbling block for his potential career as a pianist: his drenched hands slipped and struggled with the keyboard. Mother and son were desperate for an effective therapy.

I had been in practice for over a decade so it might seem surprising that this was my first encounter. In part, this was because surgical treatment for hyperhidrosis was in its infancy. It was not often performed at the time, so it was not widely known. Too, the environment plays an important role in the prevalence of hyperhidrosis. Although abnormal sweating can occur at any time, the disorder is encountered less frequently in cooler climates where there is less need for lowering body temperature, and, consequently less "background" stimulation of sweating. Moving from Chicago to the Southwest put me in the sort of hot and dry environment that made it much more likely that I would encounter patients with hyperhidrosis.

Sweat glands are ubiquitous; hyperhidrosis can affect any region of the body. My patient had palmar hyperhidrosis which affects the hands, one of the more common forms of the disease. The other most frequently involved area is the armpit, where it is referred to as axillary hyperhidrosis. The two can occur together but, as with my patient, frequently only one area is affected. Although these are the two most commonly impacted locations, the soles of the feet (plantar hyperhidrosis) and the face are other body locations which can be involved. No one knows why any particular part of the body but not another is caught up in the disease process. Wherever it manifests, the excess sweat is, at minimum, a real nuisance. The sweat both soaks and stains clothing, sometimes requiring the afflicted person to change clothes several times during a day. Constantly moist skin also predisposes the sufferer to both fungal and bacterial skin infections. As with my patient, persistently wet hands can interfere not only with professional activities but can complicate routine daily tasks such as wielding tools, handling a cell phone, and working with other electronic devices. And all these considerations are on top of the impact on social and romantic life, which can be emotionally devastating.

Even though the cause of hyperhidrosis is unknown, there are treatment alternatives. The thoracic surgical therapeutic approach is to address the problem at the level of the sympathetic nerve chain in the chest, to take away the connection between the brain and the sweat glands. The brain can fire off all the anxiety messages it wants, but if they aren't delivered to the target glands, they are ineffective. In fact, for other diseases, surgeons were operating to excise portions of the chain as early as the end of the nineteenth century. These operations were performed sporadically for a variety of unexplainable reasons—epilepsy and idiocy were two—but, as you would imagine, they never entered the surgical mainstream.

In 1935 the surgeon Adson, applying his understanding of the physiological role of the sympathetic nervous system in the sweating process, resected part of the sympathetic chain from the chest of a patient with palmar hyperhidrosis, and obtained what he called a successful outcome. This surgical undertaking, however, never became popular because the procedure could only be performed through a chest operation. As you are now well aware, this open thoracotomy entails a long incision with entry into the chest cavity gained by spreading ribs apart, exposing the patient to the gamut of risks attendant to a major operative procedure and guaranteeing considerable pain afterward. Not many surgeons or hyperhidrosis patients thought this to be a reasonable trade-off of risks and benefits. The balance between these two, however, shifted with the introduction of minimally invasive surgical techniques.

As elaborated in Chapter Seven, "minimally invasive surgery" is performed through very short incisions, in contrast to the historical surgical practice of making an incision generous enough to allow open access to the target area with unimpeded visibility and sufficient room for hands and instruments. No need for a metal retractor to spread and hold the ribs apart. That causes pain by irritating the chest wall nerves alongside the ribs; cutting the muscles of the chest wall does as well. During minimally invasive operations, small tubes called ports are placed through the cuts in the skin. This obviates both of the major causes of postoperative pain, as muscle is not sliced and there is no rib-spreading. The surgeon uses a video camera through one of the ports, and its images are displayed on several screens before the surgeon. Long operating instruments are manipulated through the other ports and used to conduct the operation. There are several benefits to this paradigm shift in how operations are performed. The stimulation to the patient's inflammatory system is less than for open operations by several orders of magnitude—so patients feel better, hurt less, and recover more quickly. In the light of these benefits, it was inevitable that thoracoscopic operations to deal with the segment of the sympathetic nerve chain that sends impulses to and controls sweating in the axilla and hand would begin. By the end of the 1990s, these were established as the operation of choice for palmar and axillary hyperhidrosis.

Regardless of the way the operation is performed, it is essential to determine the portion of the sympathetic chain that corresponds with the part of the body doing the sweating. The surgical goal is to deal only with this relevant bit of the chain. No one wants an insufficient operation but, on the other hand, taking out more chain than necessary could result in undesired consequences such as bringing normal sweating elsewhere in the body to a halt. (Remember, a certain amount is good for you.) Time and experience have allowed the development of a reasonably accurate map which correlates parts of the nerve chain with the specific body areas they control. It's not a precise map, as neural wiring always differs between individuals (just as do most of our bodily characteristics—we are not carbon copies of each other). So, we know what to go after, but definitive answers to three important questions remain. What should the surgeon do to the nerve chain; what are the results as defined by the balance among the benefits, side effects, and complications of the operation; and which patients are appropriate candidates for the surgical option?

When the patient decides on surgery, what does the surgeon do during the thoracoscopic procedure? In fact, there are technical options and a single "best" is open for debate. Many reports have accumulated in the surgical literature from multiple surgeons representing several countries using a variety of operations; however, results of the procedures, despite differences in operative techniques, are similar. One choice is to extirpate—that is, to simply remove the segment of the sympathetic chain responsible for the stimulation of the patient's sweat glands. Another approach is to use an electrocautery instrument and destroy the same length of chain with heat. The final alternative is to place metal clips at the two ends of the chain segment. All of these operations are called "sympathectomy," as all three remove the sympathetic chain either literally, by destroying it, or by isolating it so that it can't function. Not surprisingly, given that the "map" is not perfectly precise. What does differ among surgeons is the understanding of exactly how much of the nerve chain should be dealt with. The longer the excised, cauterized, or clipped segment, the more certain the excessive sweating is of being stopped, but also the more likely are side effects of the operation. A conservative surgical approach seems the most reasonable philosophy to guide the surgeon.

What are the outcomes of these operations, what do they accomplish, and what are the complications? Most importantly, they consistently and reliably stop the sweating in the previously involved part of the body. In the operating room, the hands of patients with the palmar variety become warm and dry the instant the sympathetic chain is ablated. It's instantaneous, as though a light switch were thrown. As patients wake from anesthesia and are visited by family, the improvement is immediately obvious; it's not unusual to see tears of happiness. (This gives some insight into the emotional toll the disease takes.) The results are equally as good for hyperhidrosis of the axillary and plantar locations. The operation, regardless of the operative technique the surgeon prefers, will control the sweating. But there is another side of the coin, although serious complications are rare. The surgeon can nick a blood vessel when resecting the sympathetic chain and get troublesome bleeding. This is quite uncommon and typically easily handled. Infection inside the chest is a possibility, but I am not aware of an instance being reported in the surgical literature.

There is, however, a trade-off for the elimination of sweating due to a troublesome side effect of the surgery called compensatory sweating. It's as though there were a thermostat setting for the desired sweating level in the previously affected area and once it has been excluded from the sweating loop, the brain frantically turns up sweating everywhere, seemingly to restore the level set by the thermostat for the body part where hyperhidrosis once reigned. Some patients never experience this so-called compensatory sweating; for others their back or torso begins to sweat enough to constitute a minor irritant—much less of a concern and bother than the original problem. But for a minority, the operation has simply shifted the excess sweating problem to new locations again necessitating frequent clothing changes. The exact frequency with which this unhappy complication occurs is uncertain, as the many articles in the surgical literature report a substantial range for the fraction of patients who develop compensatory sweating. Two factors play a role, one technical and one environmental. The incidence seems to be greater when the surgeon interrupts the sympathetic chain relatively high in the chest (again suggesting the prudence of surgical conservatism) and, logically, just like hyperhidrosis, compensatory sweating is more likely in warmer climates.

Reviewing the complications of thoracoscopic sympathectomy reminds me that determining the frequency and severity of complications of any operation exposes an intriguing aspect of the patient-surgeon relationship. Although most patients openly report and even complain about a less than perfect result from an operation—reasonably and appropriately—it is a well-known phenomenon that many with an untoward result are reluctant to do so. It's as though they don't want to criticize their surgeon. For this reason, when a study of the results of an operation is carried out, it is ideal to have someone other than the surgeon talk to the patient, who is more likely to be candid with, and identify complications to, a third party.

The remaining question is how to choose patients for whom this operation is appropriate. The first therapeutic step for all who sweat is not an operation but, quite reasonably, topical antiperspirants. These agents are relatively inexpensive, easy to use, readily available, and frequently suffice for patients with milder amounts of sweating, particularly for the axillary location and in cooler climates. Most agents contain a compound of aluminum which precipitates out of solution and forms a solid salt when it mixes with sweat. This salt forms a plug that blocks the duct which is the sweat conduit from the gland to the skin. The sweat is trapped inside the gland. Topical agents do not always suffice, particularly when sweating is copious enough to overwhelm the plug and push it out of the sweat gland duct. In addition to the sensibleness of beginning treatment in this fashion, it is also true that most insurance companies will not reimburse for alternative therapies until topical agents have been tried—a little real-world insight.

When the topical antiperspirants are insufficient, there are two additional non-surgical options. One is to use Botox, whose scientific name is botulinum neurotoxin, of cosmetic fame and notoriety. When injected beneath the skin, the drug blocks the transmission of nerve signals so that the stimulus from the sympathetic nerves never reaches the sweat glands; they don't go into high gear. Small needles are used so pain is not a concern when the axilla is being treated, and discomfort can be mitigated by icing the area first to obtain some numbness. The treatments are much more likely to cause pain in the hands or soles of the feet so first injecting an anesthetic to block the sensations from the major nerve(s) coming from the treated location is a kind thing to do. Botox of course, is unable to selectively block only the nerves to the sweat glands; it affects all nerves. As a result, some weakness in hand muscles is common when treating palmar hyperhidrosis. These Botox injections are efficacious, but the results are not permanent; repeat sessions are necessary every six to 18 months.

Another alternative, suitable mainly for palmar and plantar hyperhidrosis, is called "iontophoresis." It works by passing an ionized substance through the patient's intact skin. This is achieved by a mild electric current in a shallow water tray filled with simple tap water while the patient's hands or feet are fully immersed. The first few treatments are performed in a clinic with supervision but subsequently can be continued at home as needed, perhaps monthly, with the use of an iontophoresis device. Since it is not known precisely how this method works (though it is speculated the efficacy is related to a thickening of the skin), one wonders exactly why it was first attempted over a century ago. Certainly, the reason is not intuitively obvious. The answer must lie with a common early misconception that electricity contained some sort of mysterious healing property. Roughly 80% of users report their condition improved and suffer less, but still some, sweating. There are no major complications with iontophoresis although there are occasional mild shocks. I would not have liked to be an early trial patient while the right electric current was being determined. I envision a Goldilocks-like scenario as a series of patients leap, literally galvanized, from the water tray, as variable experimental shocks are delivered till one is pronounced: "just right."

There are no absolute criteria for selecting patients for surgery. As a minimum, all candidates should have given topical agents a chance to control the problematic sweating. If topical agents are insufficient, the next step, ideally, is for the patient to make an informed decision and choose for themselves among the three remaining options. Some will prefer one of the two non-surgical approaches of Botox injections or iontophoresis; for others, the operation will appeal. This is where the patient's attitudes and preferences come into play. Some are bothered by the need for repetitive injections or iontophoresis treatments and would prefer a single operation. Others who are leery of surgery, will go with one of the non-operative methods. As with surgery for GERD, surgery for this functional disorder is elective. Operations for hyperhidrosis and GERD are to control symptoms and improve someone's quality of life, not to cure a cancer.

My patient, unsatisfied with topical agents and after considering the pros and cons, wanted a sympathectomy. Since of course, he had two affected sides, I performed bilateral sympathectomies. I inserted three ports, five millimeters in diameter, through same-sized incisions on the patient's right side. The anesthesiologist used a special breathing tube to selectively ventilate only the left lung. This allowed the lung in the operated chest to collapse. This being my first sympathectomy—of course the patient was aware—I was a little apprehensive, mainly about identifying the small sympathetic chain; it's about the thickness of two or three threads together. I had read all I could find in preparation; this was before the ubiquitous videos of every minimally invasive operation, now easily found on the Internet.

Aided by the magnification offered by the surgical optical system, it was easy to spot the sympathetic chain running up and down beneath the cover of the thin, translucent, parietal pleura. I picked the pleura up like a sheet from a bed and, using scissors, cut it along the length of the chain, which I gently lifted. I cut it in two places, removing the desired segment. The anesthesiologist reported the patient's right hand warmed up immediately. After closing the small incisions, the patient was turned on his right side and the procedure repeated in his left chest. In the recovery room, tears flowed from family as he awoke. He left the hospital the next day, using only over-the-counter medications for his mild pain.

Follow-up two weeks later found him quite happy; his hands were warm and dry. At six months, his hands remained the same, but he noticed an increase in sweat on his chest and back. Yet he was content with the trade-off, as he was more comfortable in social situations, and better able to pursue his piano career. This result was consistent with my overall experience in subsequent patients: about a third noted compensatory sweating but in only a few was it sufficiently copious that they regretted their sympathectomy.

16
▼

BACK TO THE
MIDWEST

I began to chafe because of the lost opportunities in southern Nevada and became sufficiently frustrated as the potential for growth and development of the medical school there passed us by that another move became appealing. This time, it was back to the Midwest as Chair of the Surgery Department at Wright State University in Dayton, Ohio. Although the inevitable challenges were waiting, along with cold and snow, overall, this was a positive move. The academic stature of the school was stronger, the surgery residency program was larger and in good shape, and recruitment of new faculty was possible.

As for challenges, most of them were actually cleverly disguised opportunities to foster the Department's welfare. There was the inevitable resistance of the area's private surgeons to departmental growth—the town-gown bugaboo of perceived (and actual) competition, as I described encountering in Las Vegas. It's a funny thing: my experience in both Las Vegas and Dayton was that private surgeons didn't bat an eye when another private surgeon arrived in town, but it seemed to inflame them when the medical school added faculty.

The move to Ohio was stimulating. I immersed myself in doing the things I loved: teaching and interacting with students, recruiting and mentoring faculty and residents, associating with and developing friendships with the academic physicians in the school—including, but not limited to, my fellow surgeons—and continuing to see patients and practice surgery.

But the agency that accredits residency programs had mandated so many new requirements, mainly regarding the number of total hours residents could work each week as well as the number of consecutive hours, that I no longer felt I could both perform my chairman duties and be directly in charge of the residency program, as was the case in Nevada. Luckily, I had the perfect faculty member to assume that responsibility, but I missed the close association with the general surgery residents I had enjoyed in Nevada.

Surgeons all love to operate and I was no exception. Between the daunting winters that restricted outdoor activity, and the midwestern tradition of hearty eating, people in Ohio were generously proportioned, which led to a prevalence of GERD. Obesity is a known risk factor for GERD, presumably because the weight of the abdominal wall tissue (the pot-belly phenomenon) puts pressure on the abdominal cavity. This compresses the stomach and squeezes its acidic contents up into the esophagus. Surprisingly, there was not a robust local interest in the surgical treatment of GERD, a void I was happy to take advantage of. I had been interested in this disease, both its pathophysiology and its operative management, since my University of Chicago research days. I had performed a considerable number of both Belsey and Nissen antireflux procedures over the years. Relieving patients of annoying and even debilitating heartburn and regurgitation was always personally satisfying.

However, repeatedly doing these procedures had become routine, so that performing myself or leading a resident through the operation became "déjà vu all over again." The advent of minimally invasive techniques in the 90s, using a laparoscopic approach for the Nissen fundoplication, stimulated me. Having experience with open operations made it easier to master the new method, but there was definitely a learning curve—it was the same operation but with significant technical differences. There was the loss of tactile feedback from my fingers, and a very different visual perspective. During an open laparotomy, my visual orientation was above and outside the patient. Laparoscopic optics were quite different, as the camera was inside the patient at the level of the internal organs. Another difference: I was used to three-dimensional viewing with my own eyes—but the video screen was a two-dimensional presentation. Mastering the minimally invasive instruments took time and practice; practice using training kits and computer simulations, not in patients. Learning to adapt to this new way to accomplish an old operation, and then teaching it to residents, reinvigorated my enjoyment of the technical aspect of the undertaking.

I had learned and begun to use this minimally invasive approach in Nevada; I put it to frequent use in Ohio. Laparoscopic operations have been common for several decades now, including laparoscopic fundoplication, so that surgery residents learn the necessary techniques during their residency. Laparoscopy did not exist when I trained; I had to seek out early practitioners, and get tutored for my first few procedures, so that I was certain I could perform the operation safely and effectively. After laparoscopic surgery for GERD, my patients only spent one night in the hospital, noted minimal pain, and needed minimal analgesic medication when they went home. The low risk of any significant morbidity (with of course the two common side effects of mild and temporary dysphagia, and a reduced ability to belch), and the benefits of elimination of heartburn, regurgitation, and need to continue medications, plus a return to an unrestricted choice (if not amount) of food, was a real boon for patients with unrelenting GERD. These were among my most contented patients. Although an operation to control acid reflux is not as dramatic as an operation for cancer, it improves someone's quality and enjoyment of life, and that is a rewarding outcome for both patient and surgeon.

An interesting and unanticipated finding is that following a laparoscopic Nissen fundoplication, patients frequently find that their shoulders are sore for a few days. While there are other potential etiologies of this unexpected event, a likely cause is that the carbon dioxide gas used to distend the abdomen reacts with the water in the saline solution instilled by the surgeon to clear the tissues. Carbonic acid is formed by this chemical reaction and is capable of irritating the undersurface of the diaphragm. The diaphragm is driven by the phrenic nerve. As this nerve descends from the brain through the neck and chest, it sends a branch which supplies the shoulders. That is where the patient's brain assumes the discomfort is, when the nerve in the diaphragm reports encountering the acid.

My experience with patient AR was typical. This 48-year-old man had a history of many years of unrelenting heartburn, most pronounced after meals and consumption of coffee or wine. The heartburn was described by him as a burning pain starting at the lower end of his breastbone and seeming to rise upwards toward his throat. The frequency and severity were greatly diminished by his medications, but he had intermittent breakthrough occurrences if he lapsed and overate or indulged in more than a sip of coffee or wine. His major complaint now was occasional regurgitation of a bitter fluid into his mouth; this sometimes caused coughing which wakened him. He also said he worried about the need to take medications the rest of his life, and he missed the enjoyment of morning coffee and a glass of wine with dinner. Esophageal pH monitoring confirmed the diagnosis of acid reflux, and endoscopy found a small sliding hiatal hernia and ruled out a Barrett's esophagus.

We discussed the pros and cons of a laparoscopic Nissen fundoplication operation. I felt his reasons to consider this option were sufficient to proceed. I explained that the likelihood of the elimination of heartburn and regurgitation were excellent, but the tradeoff would be the need to resist large meals, as that could result in uncomfortable bloating.

We proceeded. I next saw AR in the preoperative holding area and helped to wheel him into the operating room. Once he was anesthetized, he was positioned as was my patient with achalasia: supine with legs spread and supported with stirrups. I stood between his legs and inserted the usual five ports. Enough tissue was cut or pushed aside (a technique called blunt dissection) to liberate the lower esophagus from attachments in the hiatus. Using a harmonic scalpel, a device that uses high-frequency vibrations to simultaneously cut (separate) and coagulate (control bleeding), I divided all tissue attachments and blood vessels between the stomach and the spleen so that I could move the fundus as necessary. I then sutured the hiatus closed and performed a Nissen fundoplication with the fundus wrapped around the esophagus as described in the GERD chapter.

AR went home the next morning, taking over-the-counter medications for pain relief. One week later, he was adding solid foods to an initially soft-food diet. He did notice that his left shoulder was "sore." A few days later, he called to say that his shoulder was fine but solid foods seemed to stick on the way down. I recommended he return to a soft diet until swelling around the esophagus resolved. In my office one month later, he said he was swallowing and eating normally. He was free of both heartburn and regurgitation despite no longer taking medications.

In Ohio, I continued my surgical practice, caring for patients and operating as before, but my academic priorities had evolved as the years went along. My contributions to the thoracic surgery literature shifted from publishing original articles to editing books and contributing chapters to others. As a senior participant in academia, my motivation was to facilitate the careers of the younger faculty and encourage residents to consider an academic career. I reduced my participation in societies: I continued to be engaged chiefly by serving on committees, being a discussant of presentations, and serving on panels during annual meetings. It was time to make room for the next generation to take the forefront in presenting new information.

It was also time to admit my surprise at the number of new and unexpected, even unforeseen, additions to what thoracic surgeons do and how they do it. I have repeatedly emphasized the impact of minimally invasive surgery, both laparoscopy and thoracoscopy. When this revolution in surgical technique began, most of my colleagues and I thought it was an interesting way to take out gallbladders, but never saw this radically different method of operating replacing the good old open thoracotomy and infiltrating thoracic surgery. Wrong. With all its patient benefits, it is the present and will be the future till the next disruptive technology comes along. Technically we had evolved from "surgery" millennia ago using sharp rocks to minimally invasive operations using elongated, stick-like instruments.

Another innovation affecting thoracic surgery that arose during my time was the replacement of suturing tissue together by hand by stapling devices which can be used to divide tissues or construct anastomoses. They come in many varieties. I used linear staplers, which lay down a row of six staples in a straight line and cut between the middle two, to transect the stomach while performing an esophagectomy. A similar but shorter linear stapling instrument is now the standard for cutting across bronchi and large blood vessels such as the pulmonary artery and veins. The same devices can be used to create an anastomosis or, alternatively, a circular stapler, using the identical arrangement of cutting between arrays of staples, will do the job. Stapled anastomoses take less time to perform than sewing them and are more reliable, i.e., are less likely to break down and leak any material passing through.

Considering changes in the life of thoracic surgeons, I want to emphasize too how much managed care has dramatically altered patterns of patient care. Insurance companies began to stipulate patterns of care. One was the mandate for the surgeon to obtain prior authorization to perform an operation. This requirement appears reasonable but takes time that could be spent caring for patients and frequently frustrates as the authorizer often has no familiarity with the operation proposed by an experienced thoracic surgeon. To minimize hospital costs, surgeons began to be required to get necessary tests for patients before their admission and only bring them into the hospital the day of surgery.

Similar thinking led to earlier and earlier discharge of patients after their operation. Most of these new requirements were reasonable and did bring down costs to patients and insurers, although these policies can create hardships for patients in two ways. Patients now have to arrive very early for a morning operation, and I had to send patients home after a procedure while they still hurt or were not yet fully self-reliant. Money was saved, but some patients—and their families—were stressed and occasionally required readmission to the hospital. These patterns also meant that, since patients were not admitted into the hospital until the day of their operation, frequently my residents' first meeting with them was in the preoperative holding area. With less exposure to patients preoperatively they miss learning how to evaluate new patients—including less experience wrestling with deciding if an operation is appropriate—and did not participate in preparing them for chest operations; not just medically but emotionally. This situation has to result in new surgeons being somewhat less skilled in these areas even if their operative skills are intact.

Contemplating the education and training of surgery residents brings me to reflect on my experiences in academic thoracic surgery and the myriad aspects of the merger of these two "cultures," of academia and of chest surgery. Being an academic means being embedded in a university and medical school community—students, residents, and faculty are all members. Working with residents, helping them to develop their skills and confidence, and sharing with them the pride of completing the arc of maturation as they move from neophyte to a fully trained, competent, and completely independent surgeon was enormously gratifying. They were hard-pressed to tie square knots when they began, but five short years later the general surgery residents were capable surgeons. That was where thoracic surgery residents started—having mastered the basic techniques and surgical instruments, able to use both to perform many general surgery operations yet needing to learn to apply their skills to operations in the thoracic cavity. I also needed to continue learning and adapting to new technology. I spent hours as a student and resident practicing knot-tying, only to need to learn to tie knots from a distance using instruments rather than my hands once I encountered the new minimally invasive operations.

Similarly, the role of chair provided the opportunity to mentor young faculty surgeons and watch them develop into leaders in their chosen specialties. Collaborating with colleagues to provide new understandings of pathophysiology or results of new or modified surgical techniques to help shape how surgeons care for patients, was something I felt good about. And there was always the interaction with medical students and the delight of seeing them light up with a spark of insight charged with enthusiasm as an epiphany occurred when they connected some dry clinical fact from a textbook to an actual patient scenario and saw its relevance. All this combined to make true my premonition as a medical student: both academia and thoracic surgery were cultures with people whose company I relished. Surgeons are typically strong-willed, confident, and comfortable taking charge of clinical situations. While these traits propel some of them across the line into an excessive sense of self-importance, I never found this to be typical. When controlled, these are simply appropriate and essential attributes when dealing with urgent or critical decisions. When an operative field suddenly fills with blood, or a patient unexpectedly deteriorates in the emergency room, decisions must be made quickly; you do not want a diffident or dithering surgeon to be responsible for your surgical care.

I must add that over the years of being an academic, I generally found the interaction and friendship with physicians from other specialties stimulating and enjoyable; one of the most enjoyable aspects of the academic culture. There were exceptions, as would be true for any group of people, but the majority of my colleagues had an impressive ability to problem-solve when it came to the care of complicated patients and were able to devise and carry out scientific studies to advance our understanding of physiology and disease. Although all were appropriately focused on their professional responsibilities, most also had interests and accomplishments outside of medicine that made them a pleasure to interact with over a cup of coffee in the hospital lounge as well as socially, and to learn from, both in and out of the hospital.

We all needed each other. I had long since realized the pace of development in other specialties rendered impossible to keep up with all that was being added to the understanding of diseases or their treatments. We were still members of our tribes but whereas years ago a Venn diagram of our respective specialties would have shown little overlap, now there is a significant amount.

As the recession tightened budgets and brought opportunities for development and growth of the department to a screeching halt, it seemed the time was right for letting go; I was ready to step aside. I knew I would miss many things: operating, the culture of academia, recruiting faculty, teaching, and spending time with the future of medicine in the form of residents and students. But the time had come. I had been right as a student to head toward surgery, and right as a surgical resident to veer into academic thoracic surgery; I had no regrets.

This is true not only because of my experiences as a thoracic surgeon. As I have expressed, I appreciated all my peers, in all specialties, in academia. One characteristic I respected was their willingness to serve in inner-city university hospitals, as well as the many county and city hospitals around our country. This put them on the receiving end of the stream of uninsured patients who have no alternative but to use the clinics and emergency rooms of these hospitals. This entailed a considerable commitment of time and energy, and sacrifice of income because indigent, uninsured patients don't receive health maintenance care, and are typically in worse shape than insured patients who get preventive attention. The Accountable Care Act, popularly known as "Obamacare," improved the situation for many patients who were finally able to obtain health insurance because of its provisions; as of this writing its future is uncertain.

Retirement had arrived. I remember hearing an army general tell the story of how the reality of retirement hit him. He woke at his usual time, dressed, and climbed into the back seat of his car... and it didn't go anywhere. My epiphany was to arise only to find that for the first time in many years I had no 6:30 a.m. meeting or conference to attend and no 7:30 a.m. operation to perform.

Operating and being someone's doctor are two activities that can't be done part-time. They require full-time availability. Moving to Arizona after Ohio did provide the opportunity to remain a part of academic culture. At the University of Arizona, I taught students, mentored residents and participated in clinical research projects for several years. This was gratifying, brought new friends and colleagues, and kept me connected until I finally stepped fully away. Now I admire from afar the continuing progress in the care of patients with chest diseases. The wheel never stops turning.

17

REFLECTIONS

I've emphasized the value of minimally invasive surgery. However, there is an aspect I've left unaddressed—its impact on the training of residents. Young surgeons exposed during residency to these minimally invasive procedures are replacing those trained earlier, like me, who favor traditional open-chest approaches. This younger generation represents the state-of-the-art for our specialty. But the law of unintended consequences has resulted in some unforeseen scenarios related to training programs and resident trainees.

When performing open operations, my peers and I directly contacted our patient's bodies and organs, and our fingers gave us, literally, a feeling for the strength of tissues in each body location. We could appreciate how much tugging and probing the organs, and the tissues connecting them, would safely tolerate; we have a feel for safe limits. I learned from using my hands how vigorously I could safely manipulate tissues and organs, which ones will easily separate with gentle teasing by an educated hand, and which require careful sharp dissection with scissors or scalpel to be freed up from surrounding tissues or organs. Without embarrassment, I admit that there is also a pleasurable tactile feedback from slipping one's fingers into the tissues to gently inquiring if they are safely separable. Today's residents performing minimally invasive operations derive sensory feedback

208

secondhand from surgical instruments rather than directly from their fingers. This remove from the tissues and organs diminishes the ability to gauge tissue pliability and resilience. (There are instruments with haptic capability, but they are not yet generally available.)

Beyond this is another issue. Because of the predominance of minimally invasive surgery operations, many residents currently finishing their training and entering practice have experienced only a modest number of open procedures. This is a potentially significant drawback when they, as they inevitably must, encounter a patient not suitable for a minimally invasive procedure, or need to convert from that to an open operation. Both situations occur. This can be necessitated by intraoperative bleeding, for example, that obscures vision by covering the camera lens. Additional reasons both for conversion and for choosing an open technique over a minimally invasive one at the onset of an operation include the presence of extensive internal adhesions between organs caused by infection, or prior operations which similarly hinder visibility, and the need to deal with inflamed and fragile tissue, a situation when tactile feedback is essential. These situations will continue to be encountered; it is a challenge to prepare residents to be able to deal with them. My observations are not Luddite arguments against minimally invasive technology with its many benefits; they are observations about training and educational challenges I feel must be addressed by surgical educators.

One helpful addition to the surgical curriculum has been the widespread utilization of simulation software programs and training stations that help residents—before putting their hands on patients—develop proficiency with basic surgical techniques, such as knot-tying, and familiarize themselves with the proper sequence of operative maneuvers for specific operations. Learning these skills is particularly helpful before minimally invasive operations so that the resident can concentrate on understanding the operation and is not distracted by learning to manipulate the instruments. Appreciation for the three-dimensional anatomic relationship between, for example, the pulmonary arteries and veins—seeing how they relate to each other and getting a feeling for the tissue that supports them—still must come from experiences in an open surgical field in a real patient.

Residents in training now view the operative field almost exclusively on a two-dimensional screen without depth perception. Somewhat compensating for this handicap is that this generation of trainees grew up playing video games and texting, enhancing their dexterity. These activities are ideal practice for the challenge of mastering minimally invasive surgery. The surgical instruments for minimally invasive procedures are 18 or more inches long—much like a long stick with a grasper mechanism or a scissor at the tip—so that maneuvering them at a distance in the operative field with visualization on a flat-screen requires more, or at least different, dexterity than wielding a short scalpel with one's fingers under direct vision. Figure 9 contrasts a typical instrument used in open surgery for clamping a structure with the much longer surgical clamp used in minimally invasive operations such as laparoscopy or thoracoscopy. For scale, a 15-centimeter (approximately six-inch) ruler is shown. (Imagine the challenge of manipulating the long stick, inserted through a small hole in a screen which obstructs direct view, using visualization obtained on a TV screen, making depth indiscernible.)

So far, we have been exploring what is now considered routine, minimally invasive surgery; it has an extensive track record of safety and efficacy. An even more recent alternative to surgeons holding the instruments in their hands is the so-called surgical robotic system. "So-called" because there is not truly a robot involved. The surgeon sits at a computer console used to control mechanical "arms" which grasp and manipulate minimally invasive instruments which are inserted into the patient's abdomen or chest through the usual ports. An advantage of the robotic system is that a three-dimensional view is provided on the computer console screen from a camera system which uses *two* optic channels; this ensures the operator has a sense of depth. The robot has other helpful attributes such as the capability of rotating the tip of the instruments; its use in minimally invasive procedures is vigorously touted by some general thoracic surgeons. However, I feel some proponents are overzealous so that, in procrustean fashion, all their operations are made to fit this technology. Substituting the robot for standard laparoscopic and thoracoscopic equipment substantially increases the cost of operations; it is a quite expensive investment for a hospital. In addition,

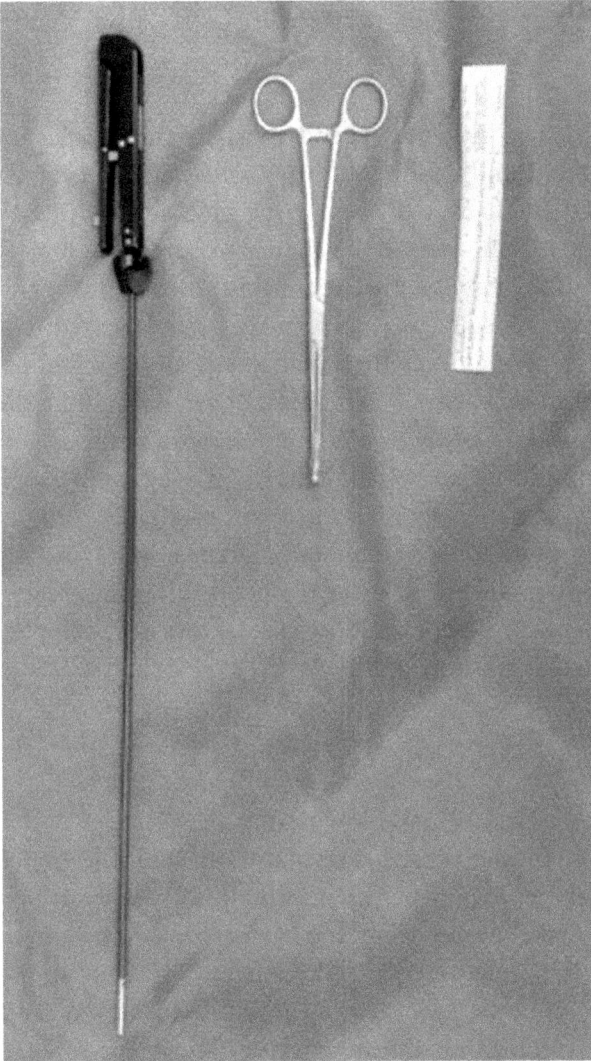

FIGURE 9.

robotic operations typically take a longer time to perform than the usual minimally invasive ones, due to the relatively complex setup required in the operating room. Finally, results of robotic operations have been reported as being as good as but not better than open ones. Therefore, despite the enthusiasm of some surgeons, I see an uncertain future for this technology.

General thoracic surgeons spend most of their time and energy thinking about and dealing with patients with lung or esophageal cancer. As dismal a way to spend time as you may think this is, the saving grace is that we have the chance to cure most of our patients. I certainly didn't cure all my patients but since I only operated when the cancer was localized, i.e., it had not metastasized, cure was at least possible. Sometimes these patients with localized cancer had been found in an early stage because of screening high-risk people for lung cancer, or of the use of endoscopy in patients with GERD, who were found to have small cancers in a Barrett's esophagus, or in follow-up of patients with known, but originally benign, Barrett's which progressed into malignancy. I repeat my constant refrain: the chance to eradicate a cancer is a good thing so screening at-risk patients makes sense but avoiding risk factors or developing preventive measures is the holy grail.

What will be the next surgical revolution to enter the arena? I'm sure incremental improvements in minimally invasive surgical instruments will make thoracoscopy and laparoscopy even more successful. Current robotic platforms may take over. But these improvements are not revolutionary; something new would be required for that term to be valid: I imagine an army of nanoscopic robots, properly programmed, and with cutting and coagulating lasers, being fed into the chest, scurrying about to complete operations. Perhaps they will be outfitted with cancer sensors to help the surgeon decide what stays and what goes. Why not?

Without question, interacting with patients was always the high point of my time as a surgeon, from meeting them in the office, to performing operations to eradicate cancer or improve the quality of life, through postoperative follow-up. It is a remarkable experience to be able to welcome a patient back from what Virginia Woolf termed "the undiscovered countries" of illness to resume their place in "the army of the upright." To know your efforts improved the quality of someone's life, or contributed to the cure of their cancer, makes worthwhile the long days, and the night visits to the emergency room or intensive care unit. Positive results also help compensate for the times when an operation does not succeed—but the stings of those failures linger and are never shrugged off. Actually curing a patient's cancer is an experience my colleagues in medical oncology share less frequently at present although the future of cancer treatment is with them. Improved, hopefully curative, or even preventive therapies will come about as a result of a combination of more efficacious chemotherapy agents, drugs targeting and disrupting specific neoplastic metabolic pathways, and genetic manipulations (although the latter, it seems, will be challenged by both ethical and political dilemmas). Men and women wielding knives will be in less demand and chests will rarely need to be cracked.

Appendix One

Glossary

The Glossary contains medical, surgical, and anatomic terms used in the book with which the reader may not be familiar. They are used in the text to describe the details of specific operative procedures and surgical techniques. In some instances, there is overlap or redundancy in the definitions and in their usage, both in the book and in the surgical community. The anatomic structures listed are displayed and identified in Appendices Two and Three.

Medical and Surgical Terms

ANASTOMOSIS: This is the joining together of two tubular anatomic organs to place them in continuity, so they have a common lumen or channel. An example of this is the suturing together of the ends of two segments of intestine after a portion has been resected, frequently to remove a cancer. Similarly, an anastomosis rejoining cut ends of a bronchus or blood vessel may be performed, and an anastomosis connecting the esophagus to the stomach is necessary following an esophagectomy. Anastomoses were historically constructed by sewing or suturing the tissues together. Since the advent of modern stapling devices, this classic technique has been in large part supplanted by this modern alternative, which has increased security by diminishing any tendency of an anastomosis not to heal properly and be watertight. The most dreaded complication of an anastomosis is for it to partly dehisce (separate) so that the contents of the approximated structures begin to leak out into a body cavity. Since the gastrointestinal tract contains bacteria, a leak from a gastrointestinal anastomosis rapidly initiates a devastating infectious process.

BOLUS: The technical name for a swallowed mass of food. Doesn't sound too tasty though.

CARCINOGEN: A substance which can cause cancer to develop.

CARCINOGENIC: Capable of causing cancer.

DEBRIDEMENT: The process of removing necrotic or infected tissues from an open wound. This is done with a knife or scissors until only healthy tissue remains. If this material is allowed to remain, a wound cannot begin to heal and is prone to become infected.

DEHISCENCE: The coming apart of a surgical incision or an anastomosis. This may happen because of tension on the two sides pulling them apart, an inadequate blood supply to keep the tissues alive, or poor surgical technique.

DYSPHAGIA: Difficulty swallowing, from the Greek *dys* "with difficulty" and *phagia* "to eat." The difficulty may be in emptying food from the mouth; may be due to blockage from any cause anywhere down the esophagus, such as cancer or a stricture; or caused by an esophageal dysmotility disorder such as achalasia.

ENDOTRACHEAL TUBE: A tube placed through the mouth into the trachea and used to ventilate (breath for) a patient.

IATROGENIC: Caused by the diagnosis, manner, or treatment of a physician. An infection after an operation is an iatrogenic complication.

INTUBATE: To place a tube in an anatomic location. Most frequently it refers to placing a breathing tube in the trachea. The tube is referred to as an endotracheal tube.

FISTULA: An abnormal passageway connecting two hollow organs or between a hollow organ and the skin. An anal fistula runs between the interior of the anus and the skin.

LIGATE: To tie an anatomic structure together, as when a blood vessel is ligated to keep it from bleeding after being cut. The suture material used for this is called the ligature.

LUMEN: The interior of a tubular organ such as a blood vessel, the trachea, and bronchial tubes, or the esophagus.

PATHOPHYSIOLOGY: This is the term used to describe the process by which a bodily organ or system fails or does not function normally. When this occurs, an individual is usually affected by the malfunction and develops related symptoms.

PHYSIOLOGY: The description of normal function and activities of our body or any of its organs.

PLICATION: The act or process of folding a bodily tissue into a new position and securing it in place, typically with sutures.

STOMA: From the Greek for "mouth," this is a surgically created permanent opening in a structure. The most typical location is the skin of the anterior surface of the abdomen. Two common examples are a colostomy, which is constructed to relieve an obstruction; and a gastrostomy, when a tube is inserted through the skin and into the stomach to be used to provide nutrition if the patient is unable to eat normally.

Anatomic Terms

AXILLA: The armpit. It contains fat, lymph nodes, and the blood vessels and nerves to and from the arm.

BRONCHUS: The two tubular extensions from the trachea which splits into a left and a right main stem bronchus to supply the two lungs. Inside the lungs the bronchi continue to branch and "arborize" (make a tree-like pattern), forming a network inside the lungs through which flows inhaled and exhaled air.

CERVICAL: Of or related to the neck. It also can indicate the cervix of the uterus but its use in this book is always the neck definition.

FASCIA: A band or sheath of connective tissue supporting or binding parts of the body. For example, there are fascia enveloping all muscles.

GASTRIC: Related to or of the stomach.

HILUM: The anatomic bundle of blood vessels and bronchi that connect the lungs to the heart and trachea. The specific structures within the hilum are the pulmonary artery, carrying blood from the heart to the lungs, the two pulmonary veins, returning blood with oxygen from the lungs back to the heart, and the main stem bronchus.

MEDIASTINUM: The territory inside the chest that harbors the structures in the middle of the chest. It is between the two lungs and contains the heart, the trachea, and the esophagus.

NEURON: A nerve cell.

PERITONEUM: A thin membrane that lines the inside of the abdominal cavity. The abdominal cavity is, therefore, occasionally referred to as the peritoneal cavity.

PHARYNX: The area in the back of the throat behind the tongue. Both the trachea and the esophagus arise from the pharynx and their openings are adjacent to each other, making it possible for pharyngeal contents to occasionally be aspirated into the trachea.

PLEURA: There are four pleurae, two in each chest. The parietal pleura is a thin membrane that lines the inside of each chest cavity so that the chest cavity is occasionally referred to as the pleural cavity. The visceral pleura is an identical membrane which forms the outer cover of each lung. These two pleural surfaces in each chest touch as the chest expands and contracts with normal breathing. As the parietal pleura secretes a small amount of fluid, this lubrication facilitates the movement of the lungs within the chest cavity.

PULMONARY: Related to or of the lungs.

SYMPATHETIC CHAIN OF NERVES: The "chain" is a stretched-out line of neurons adjacent to and parallel to the spine. Among other functions, it transmits to the body signals from the brain that control the amount of sweating.

THORAX: This is the chest. It is derived from the Greek *thorak* meaning breast plate.

TRACHEA: The tubular structure which originates in the pharynx and constitutes the passageway for air to pass in and out of the lungs. At its origin are the vocal cords which function to create speech but also protect against the aspiration of pharyngeal contents into the trachea and the lungs. The trachea bifurcates within the mediastinum into the two main stem bronchi which pass through the hilum to communicate with the lungs.

Suffixes

These are appended to the name of the anatomic area where the activity occurs:

-CENTESIS: This follows the name of a cavity and indicates its puncture with a needle or a catheter to remove fluid. A thoracentesis is removal of fluid from the thorax. This procedure is most frequently performed to identify the nature of the fluid, e.g., to determine if it is infected.

-ECTOMY: This suffix identifies an operation to remove an organ or other anatomic structure. For example, a pneumonectomy is the removal of an entire lung, while a lobectomy is the removal of the part of a lung identified as a lobe.

-OSCOPY: The precise meaning is that a camera is being used to view the inside of a body cavity. Its usage has become more inclusive and now also designates the minimally invasive procedure for which the camera is providing a video image. Examples are laparoscopy for a minimally invasive operation in the abdomen, and similarly thoracoscopy for chest procedures.

-OSTOMY: This suffix indicates that either a side or end opening in an internal organ such as the colon is sutured to the skin to create a stoma on the skin, i.e., a colostomy. Another common example is a tracheostomy.

-OTOMY: This designates the creation of an incision or opening by cutting into an anatomic structure. An example is the creation of an opening in the side of the stomach, a gastrotomy, which could then be sutured to a stoma in the abdominal wall to create a gastrostomy. A thoracotomy is an incision into the chest and a laparotomy (lap from the Greek *lapara* for flank or abdomen) is an incision into the abdomen.

-PEXY: This suffix designates the fixation of one organ or anatomic structure to another or simply the securing of one or the other in place. When a gastrostomy is created, the stomach is sutured to the underside of the abdominal wall (a gastropexy) to help support it and minimize the possibility of the stomach pulling loose from the skin. Since an antireflux operation can involve suturing the stomach either to the esophagus or to itself, it could also be termed a gastropexy.

-PLASTY: This suffix indicates that a patient's tissue is being surgically rearranged. An operation for gastroesophageal reflux disease requires altering the normal relationship between the esophagus and the stomach so that, as described in the text, part of the stomach is wrapped around the bottom of the esophagus. This is a gastroplasty.

Prefixes

ESOPHAGO-: This prefix identifies the esophagus.

GASTRO-: This prefix designates the stomach. Examples of its use are above.

MYO-: This prefix refers to muscle, so a myotomy is the cutting of a muscle.

Appendix Two

Chest Anatomy

The figures below show the relationship between the chest organs. This is not what the surgeon sees when the chest is entered to perform an operation. The esophagus lurks deep inside the mediastinum, covered by several layers of tissue: the visceral pleura, fat, lymphatic tissue, and the fibrous tissue that binds them together. The pulmonary arteries and veins are encased within the hilum as they enter or leave the heart and, moving peripherally, disappear into the lung. Careful dissection is required to expose these structures.

FIGURE 10A: This depiction of the chest or thorax shows how the rib cage and sternum (breastbone; shown in outline) constitute the bony outer framework of the chest. This hard shell (think exoskeleton but covered with muscle and skin) shelters and protects the internal thoracic organs from penetrating and blunt force trauma.

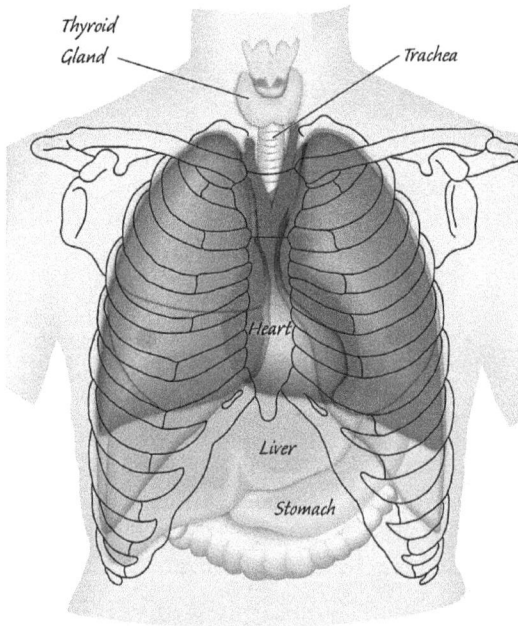

FIGURE 10A.

The lungs are the dominant internal structure. They surround and, in their normal state of full expansion, cover and hide from view the other organs, although the heart and its great vessels can be glimpsed between the two lungs. When operating in the chest, to provide access to other organs such as the esophagus and sufficient visibility to identify anatomic structures, the lung must either be gently pushed away or its elastic tissue components allowed to shrink it by the technique of only ventilating the opposite lung.

FIGURE 10B: This view is of the chest organs from the front. The trachea is descending from the pharynx (the back of the throat) and branching into a left and a right main stem bronchus, one for each lung. These two bronchi are the conduits for delivery of air with its oxygen to the lungs during inhalation, and for exhalation of gases, mainly carbon dioxide, when we exhale. The lungs are shown pulled back and partially excavated so that details of their blood vessels running through the hilum can be seen. The pulmonary artery arises from the heart and carries to the lungs the blood that has completed its circuit of the body where it surrendered its oxygen to the tissues. The pulmonary veins return to the heart the same blood after it has

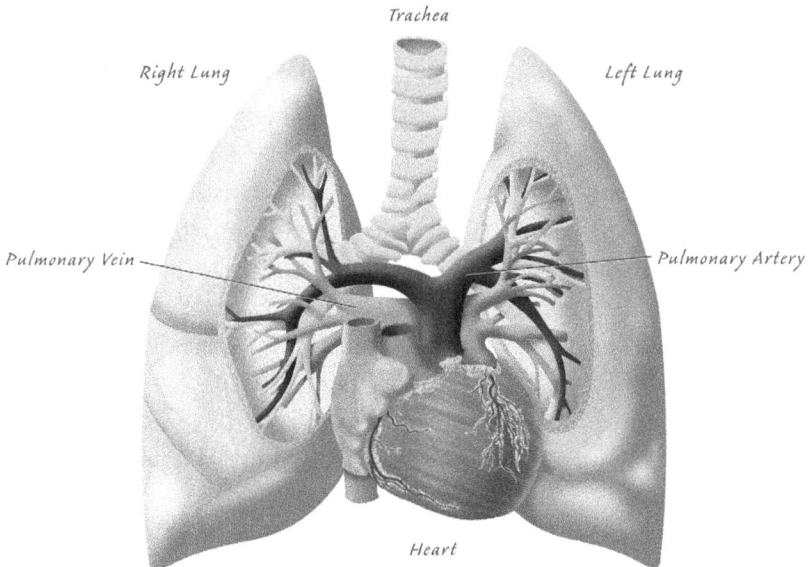

Trachea

Right Lung

Left Lung

Pulmonary Vein

Pulmonary Artery

Heart

FIGURE 10B.

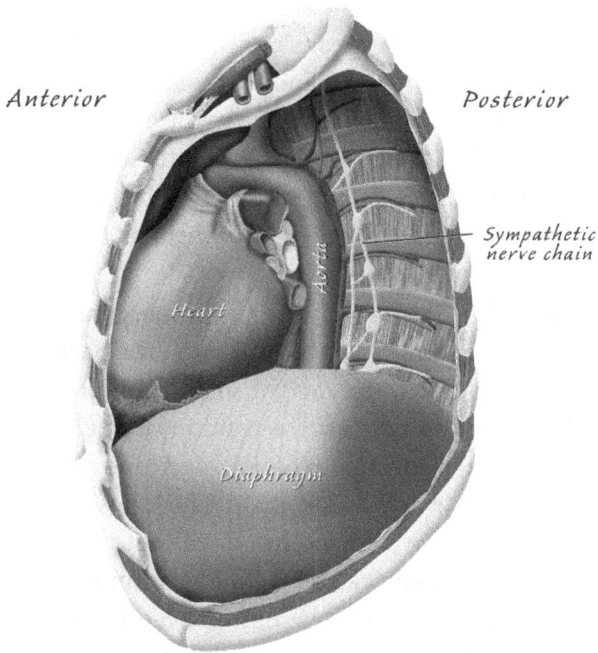

Figure 10C.

had its oxygen levels restored in its circuit through the lungs. The heart will then pump this oxygenated blood out through the aorta to the network of arteries and capillaries of the body.

FIGURE 10C: This is the inside of the left chest viewed from the side. The lungs have been removed so that the mediastinum (the central portion of the chest between the two lungs) is visible. Prominent features include the heart which is inside the pericardium (the membrane that surround and cradles it), the aorta (the large artery that leaves the heart, headed out to the body with its supply of oxygenated blood), and the origins of the pulmonary arteries and veins. The esophagus is not labeled but can be glimpsed above the aortic arch and again between the heart and aorta just above the diaphragm, the muscle that provides most of the breathing effort and separates the chest from the abdomen. The sympathetic nerves of the chest innervate the thorax, head, and arms. These nerves control some of the involuntary actions of the body, such as sweating and the contraction or dilation of blood vessels in reaction to heat or cold.

Appendix Three

Esophageal Anatomy and Physiology

Anatomy

The esophagus is a small tubular structure, only roughly an inch in diameter when maximally stretched. It has no rigidity; rather, it is quite supple. It is usually collapsed but is pliant and distensible so that it stretches open to accommodate swallowed material. It has an inner lining, called the mucosa, of squamous epithelium which is almost identical to and has many of the same characteristics as skin. Moving from inside out, past the mucosa are two muscular layers. The innermost muscle fibers are oriented in a circular fashion while the fibers of the outer muscular layer are in a longitudinal orientation. These muscles are not under volitional control; they react involuntarily to several stimuli, particularly a swallow. There are small glands imbedded in the wall just beneath the mucosa which secrete a small amount of mucous into the inside or lumen, presumably for lubrication to aid the passage of swallowed food, especially poorly chewed and hastily swallowed bits.

FIGURE 11A: This is the course of the esophagus as it descends through the chest. It begins in the neck, originating at the back of the pharynx, behind the mouth and tongue. The pharynx is a common chamber from which both the esophagus and the trachea (windpipe) to the lungs arise. When we swallow, the muscles of the pharynx fold over a tissue flap called the "epiglottis" to cover the entrance into the trachea, called the "glottis." This prevents food or drink from being aspirated into the airway during the swallowing process. (As emphasized below, when aspiration does occur, an airway reflex stimulates vigorous coughing to expel the material.) When we are not eating or swallowing saliva, a muscle deep within the neck which surrounds the esophagus remains contracted to close it, thus both preventing air from entering the esophagus with each breath, and esophageal

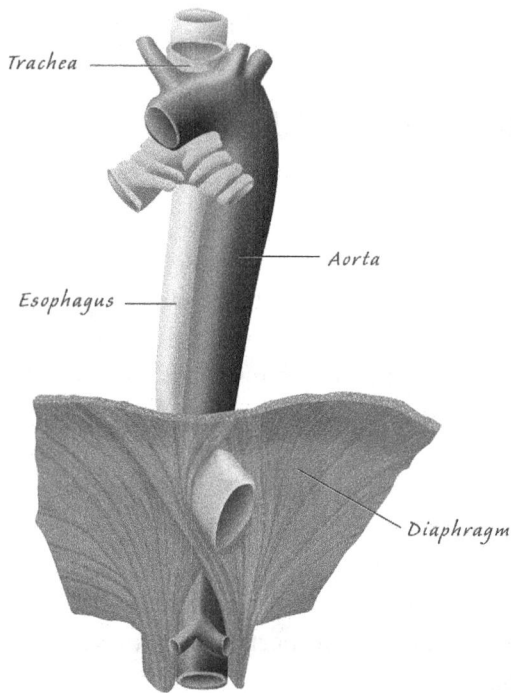

FIGURE 11A.

contents from regurgitating into the pharynx. This muscle band is termed the upper esophageal sphincter.

Moving down into the chest from the neck, the esophagus traverses the chest in a posterior location. It lies on the spine behind the heart and nestles adjacent to the aorta. Its destination is the stomach in the abdomen. To reach the stomach, the esophagus must penetrate the diaphragm, the muscular band which partitions the chest from the abdomen and is responsible for most of the work of breathing. Passage through the diaphragm takes place through the esophageal hiatus, a triangularly shaped opening adjacent to the aortic hiatus, a separate gap which allows the aorta to transit the diaphragm. Once below the diaphragm, usually for a distance of several centimeters (so that there is a significant length inside the positive pressure environment of the abdomen), the esophagus enters the stomach. There is no obvious muscle band in this location; however, the arrangement and pattern of the muscle layers of the esophagus and stomach where the two come together create a lower esophageal sphincter, a high-pressure zone, which has a constant tonic pressure. This constant squeeze prevents stomach acid from refluxing from the stomach and gaining access to the esophagus and causing symptoms ranging from occasional heartburn to true GERD, a disease discussed in the book. As with the upper esophageal sphincter, the lower sphincter must relax with swallowing to allow the solid or liquid contents to pass into the stomach.

Physiology

The sole function of the esophagus is to transport food from the mouth to the stomach where true digestion begins. This is not a passive process in which gravity does all the work. In fact, were you so inclined (literally), you could effectively swallow while hanging by your knees.

Figure 11B: This image depicts a motility study which is performed to assess esophageal function. I performed this exam in many patients during my research year at the University of Chicago. To the left is the esophagus with the stomach at the bottom. A catheter is inside the esophagus after I slipped it through the patient's nose. The catheter has pressure sensors at multiple levels inside the esophagus including the lower esophageal sphincter (LES). A swallow sets off a pressure wave—a series of contractions—which moves down the esophagus. As the wave passes each sensor it is detected and measured by the height of the "spike" on the motility tracing to the right. The sequential progress of the contractions from top to bottom—which takes only a few seconds—means they are peristaltic; they will propel food toward the stomach. The lowest tracing comes from the pressure sensor in the LES and shows it relaxing as it should.

The process of swallowing to clear the mouth begins after the teeth have macerated the food and the food has mixed with saliva to create a bolus. The muscles of the pharynx coordinate with the tongue to propel the food bolus toward the opening into the esophagus as the epiglottis folds over and guards the trachea. (When anything other than air enters the trachea, it is called "aspiration,"

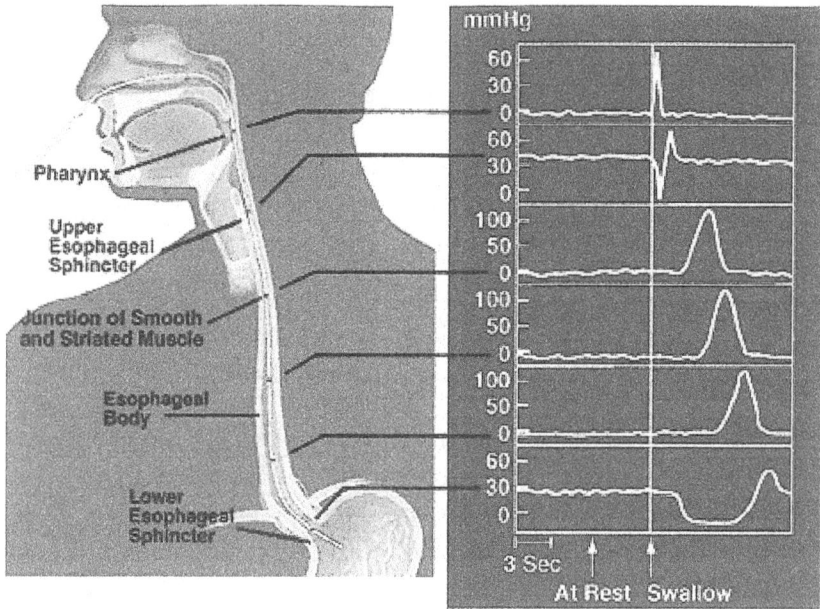

FIGURE 11B.

and can lead to pneumonia if sufficient contamination of the lung occurs. Not surprisingly, aspiration induces a vigorous coughing reflex to clear the material.) Simultaneously with swallowing, the upper esophageal sphincter relaxes, which allows the bolus to enter the esophagus, and then the sphincter resumes its resting tone to prevent regurgitation.

Swallowing also initiates a series of contractions of the muscle of the esophageal body. These contractions are peristaltic: they are sequential from top to bottom, and propel the food bolus toward the stomach, where it encounters an already relaxed lower esophageal sphincter. This seemingly premature relaxation allows the passage of liquids; their lubricating action allows them to arrive sooner than solids due to gravity speeding them along. The sphincter remains relaxed until the peristaltic wave has arrived, allowing the bolus to enter the stomach, and then regains its tone to retard gastroesophageal reflux. When the contractions are weak or occur simultaneously, they are incapable of efficacious food transport and the patient experiences difficulty swallowing, i.e., has dysphagia. Similarly, dysphagia results when either of the two sphincters malfunction and doesn't relax appropriately to allow passage of a food bolus. As emphasized in the chapter on the surgical treatment of GERD, having a length of the esophagus within the abdominal cavity is important in the normal or physiologic prevention of acid reflux. This anatomic positioning ensures that any pressure generated within the abdomen, say by straining to cough or having a bowel movement, will be equally applied to the esophagus as to the stomach, canceling any tendency to "squeeze" gastric acid up into the esophagus.

Bibliography

General

These books are excellent resources for an overview of the development of many surgical activities, especially surgery of the chest. They identify many of the early thoracic surgeons and explore their contributions to the origin and development of chest surgery.

The articles are from professional journals, with one exception. Their scope is not as wide as the books, but they also provide insight into the broad development and history of thoracic surgery.

Brewer, Lyman A. "History of Surgery of the Esophagus," *American Journal of Surgery* 139 (1980): 730-743.

Eloesser, L. "Milestones in Thoracic Surgery," *Journal of Thoracic and Cardiovascular Surgery* 60 (1970): 157-165.

Graham, Evarts A. "A Brief Account of the Development of Thoracic Surgery and Some of Its Consequences," *Surgery, Gynecology and Obstetrics* 104 (1956): 241-250.

Hochberg, Lew A. *Thoracic Surgery Before the 20th Century.* New York: Vantage Press, 1960.

Hurt, Raymond. *The History of Cardiothoracic Surgery from Early Times.* New York: Pantheon Publishing Group, 1966.

Meade, Richard H. *A History of Thoracic Surgery.* Springfield, IL: Charles C. Thomas, 1961.

Naef, Andreas P. *The Story of Thoracic Surgery.* Toronto: Hogrefe and Huber, 1990.

Ochsner, Alton. "History of Thoracic Surgery," *Surgical Clinics of North America* 46 (1966): 1355-1376.

Paget, Stephen. *The Surgery of the Chest.* London: John Wright, 1896.

Rienhoff, Jr., William F. "Twenty-Five Years' Progress in Diagnosis and Surgical Treatment of Common Chest Conditions," *American Surgeon* 21 (1955): 653-662.

Focused

Some of these books are about something other than surgery but most are focused on a particular topic or surgeon. They provide insight into the personalities and motives of individual surgeons and give depth to their lives and contributions. Many also place surgeons in the context of their society and culture. The circumstances around the introduction of new thinking by the pioneering thoracic surgeons and their operations are explored. Others concern themselves with a specific time and era of surgery.

The articles address the contributions of a single surgeon or the activity of the panoply of surgeons who contributed to the surgical struggles with a specific disease, or to the development and refinement of a new thoracic surgical technique or operation.

Chapter One

Gladwell, Malcolm. *Outliers*. New York: Little, Brown, 2010.

Norman, Geoffrey. "Winnersville USA," *Sports Illustrated*, October 1, 1988.

Saint- Exupéry, Antoine de. *The Little Prince*. Translated by Richard Howard. New York: Harcourt, 1943.

Chapter Two

Bishop, W.J. *The Early History of Surgery*. New York: Barnes and Noble Books, 1960.

Brill, Jason B., Evan K. Harrison, Michael J. Sise and Romeo C. Ignacio, Jr. "The History of the Scalpel," *Bulletin of the American College of Surgeons*103 (2018): 34-39.

Churchill, E.D., R.H. Sweet, L. Soutter and J.G. Scannell. "The Surgical Management of Carcinoma of the Lung," *Journal of Thoracic Surgery* 20 (1950): 349-365.

Gawande, Atul. "Two Hundred Years of Surgery," *New England Journal of Medicine* 366 (2012): 1716-1723.

Jungraithmayr, W. and W. Weder. "Chest Surgical Disorders in Ancient Egypt: Evidence of Advanced Knowledge," *Annals of Surgery* 255 (2012): 605-608.

Meade, Richard H. *An Introduction to the History of General Surgery.* Philadelphia: W.B. Saunders, 1968.

Moore, Wendy. *The Knife Man.* New York: Broadway Books, 2005.

Nicholl, Charles. *Leonardo da Vinci. Flights of the Mind.* New York: Viking Penguin, 2004.

Ochsner, John. "The Surgical Knife," *Bulletin of the American College of Surgeons* 84 (1999): 27-31.

Power, D.A., and Liston, Robert. *Dictionary of National Biography.* London: Smith, Elder, 1909.

Sheldon, George F. "To the Shade of John Hunter: Philip Syng Physick of Philadelphia, 'The Father of American Surgery,' Hunter's Favorite American Trainee," *Journal of the American College of Surgeons* 215 (2012): 731-736.

Tilney, Nicholas L. *Invasion of the Body.* Cambridge, MA: Harvard University Press, 2011.

Chapter Four

Naef, A.P. "The Mid-Century Revolution in Thoracic and Cardiovascular Surgery: Part 3," *Interactive Cardiovascular and Thoracic Surgery* 3 (2004): 3-10.

Macewen, William. "The Cavendish Lecture: Some Points in the Surgery of the Lung," *British Medical Journal* 2 (1906): 3-7.

Ochsner, Alton. "The Development of Pulmonary Surgery, with Special Emphasis on Carcinoma and Bronchiectasis," *American Journal of Surgery* 135 (1978): 732-746. Williams, Harley.

Chapter Five

Belsey, Ronald. "On the Teaching of Operative Surgery," *West England Medical Journal* 105 (1990): 102, 122.

Chapter Six

Davison, M.H. Armstrong. *The Evolution of Anesthesia.* Altrinchain, UK: John Sherrott and Son, 1965.

Findlen, Paula. "A History of the Lungs," Course Material, History

13 /HPS 115, The Emergence of Medicine: Middle Ages and the Renaissance. Accessed November 10, 2019. Stanford.edu/class/history13/earlysciencelab/body/lungspages/lung.

Gray, Laman. *The Life and Times of Ephraim McDowell.* Danville, KY: Ephraim McDowell House, 1987.

Keys, Thomas E. *The History of Surgical Anesthesia.* New York: Dover, 1945.

Snow, Stephanie J. *Blessed Days of Anaesthesia.* Oxford: Oxford University Press, 2008.

Wynn, Jake. "Beyond Consciousness and Pain: Dr. Morton and Anesthesia at the Battle of Spotsylvania," *Blog,* National Museum of Civil War Medicine, May 10, 2018. www.civilwarmed.org/spotsylvania/.

Chapter Seven

American Lung Association. Diagnosing and treating tuberculosis.www.lung-health-and-diseases/lung-diseases-lookup/tuberculosis/diagnosing-and-treating-tuberculosis.html.

Carter, K. Codell. Scott Abbott and James L. Siebach. "Five Documents Relating to the Final Illness and Death of Ignaz Semmelweis," *Bulletin of the History of Medicine* 69 (1995): 255-270.

D'Amours, Ray H., Frank X. Riegler, Alex G. Little. "Pathogenesis and Management of Persistent Post-Thoracotomy Pain," *Surgical Clinics of North America* 8 (1998);703-722.

Lane, Hilary J., Nava Blum and Elizabeth Fee. "Oliver Wendell Holmes and Ignaz Philipp Semmelweis: Preventing the Transmission of Puerperal Fever," *American Journal of Public Health* 100 (2010): 1008-1009.

Nakayama, Don K. "The Poet, His Poem, and the Surgeon: The Stories Behind the Enduring Appeal of 'Invictus,'" *Journal of Surgical Education* 72 (2014): 170-175.

Park, Bernard J. "Is Surgical Morbidity Decreased with Minimally Invasive Lobectomy?" *The Cancer Journal* 2011; 17:18-22.

Rutkow, Ira. "Joseph Lister and His 1876 Tour of America," *Annals of Surgery* 257 (2013): 1181-1187.

Pomerantz, Benjamin J., Joseph C. Cleveland, Heather K. Olson, Marvin Pomerantz. "Pulmonary Resection for Multi-Drug Resistant Tuberculosis," *Journal of Thoracic and Cardiovascular Surgery* 121 (2001): 448-453.

Wood, William Barry. "The Use of Antibiotics in the Treatment of Bacterial Infections," *Laryngoscope* 57 (1947): 657-663.

Chapter Nine

Allison, P.R. "Reflux Esophagitis, Sliding Hiatal Hernia, and the Anatomy of Repair," *Surgery, Gynecology and Obstetrics* 92 (1951): 414-431.

Beaumont, William. *Experiments and Observations on the Gastric Juice and the Physiology of Digestion.* Plattsburgh, NY: F.P. Allen, 1833.

Belsey, Ronald. "Stainless Steel Wire Suture Technique in Thoracic Surgery," *Thorax* 1 (1946): 39-47.

Belsey, R., K. Dowlatshahi, G. Keen and D.B. Skinner. "Profound Hypothermia in Cardiac Surgery," *Journal of Thoracic and Cardiovascular Surgery* 56 (1968): 497-509.

Fults, D.W. and P. Taussky. "The Life of Rudolf Nissen: Advancing Surgery Through Science and Principle," *World Journal of Surgery;* 35 (2011): 1402-1408.

Jeyasingham, Kumarasingham and Toni Lerut. "In Memoriam: Ronald Herbert Robert Belsey," *Diseases of the Esophagus* 21 (2008): 193-194.

Liebermann-Meffert, Dorothea and Hubert J. Stein. *Rudolf Nissen and the World Revolution of Fundoplication.* Heidelberg: Johann Ambrosius Booth Verlag, 1999.

Little, Alex G. "Mechanisms of Action of Antireflux Surgery," *World Journal of Surgery* 16 (1992): 320-325.

Morgagni, G.B.. *The Seats and Causes of Diseases Investigated by Anatomy* (1749). Translated by Benjamin Alexander. Birmingham, AL: Gryphon, 1983.

Naef, A.P. "The Mid-Century Revolution in Thoracic and Cardiovascular Surgery: Part 3," *Interactive Cardiovascular and Thoracic Surgery* 3 (2004): 3-10.

National Institute of Diabetes and Digestive and Kidney Diseases. "Digestive Diseases Statistics for the United States." Health Information. Health Statistics. Accessed November 10, 2019. www. niddk.nih.gov/health-information/health-statistics/digestive-diseases.

Nissen, Rudolf. "Gastropexy and 'Fundoplication' in Surgical Treatment of Hiatal Hernia." *American Journal of Digestive Diseases* 10 (1961): 954-961.

Skinner, David B. and Ronald H.R. Belsey. "Surgical Management of Esophageal Reflux and Hiatus Hernia: Long Term Results with 1,030 Patients," *Journal of Thoracic and Cardiovascular Surgery* 53 (1967): 33-54.

Turk, Robert P., and Alex G. Little. "The History of Surgery for Hiatal Hernia and Gastroesophageal Reflux Disease." In *Gastroesophageal Reflux Disease: Principles of Disease, Diagnosis and Treatment,* edited by F.A. Grandroth, T. Kamolz and R. Pointer, 159-165. Austria: Springer Verlag, 2006.

University of Florida Health. "Gastroesophageal Reflux Disease." Accessed November 10, 2019. https://ufhealth.org/gastroesophageal-reflux-disease.

Zhao, Y. and W. Encinosa. "Gastroesophageal Reflux Disease (GERD) Hospitalizations in 1998 and 2005: Statistical Brief [[#]]44." In *Healthcare Cost and Utilization Project (HCUP) Statistical Briefs [Internet].* Rockville, MD: Agency for Healthcare Research and Quality (US), January 2008. https://www.ncbi.nlm.nih.gov/books/NBK56308/.

Chapter Ten

Cash, Brooks D. and Roy K.H. Wong. "Historical Perspective of Achalasia," *Gastrointestinal Endoscopy Clinics of North America* 11 (2001): 221-233.

Laskowski, Igor A., Warren D. Widmann and Mark A. Hardy. "Eponymous Surgeon: Who and What Was Mikulicz," *Current Surgery* 61 (2004): 301-306.

Little, Alex G., Arturo Soriano, Mark K. Ferguson, Charles S. Winans and David B. Skinner. "Surgical Treatment of Achalasia: Results with

Esophagomyotomy and Belsey Repair," *Annals of Thoracic Surgery* 45 (1988): 489-494.

Payne, W. Spencer. "Heller's Contribution to the Surgical Treatment of Achalasia of the Esophagus," *Annals of Thoracic Surgery* 48 (1989): 876-81.

Willis, Thomas. *Pharmaceutice Rationalis Diatriba de Medicamentorum Operationibus in Humano Corpore.* London, 1674.

Zajaczkowski, Thaddaeus. "Johann Anton von Mikulicz-Radecki: A Pioneer of Gastroscopy and Modern Surgery," *World Journal of Urology* 26 (2008): 75-86.

Chapter Eleven

Ludlow, Abraham. "A Case of Obstructed Deglutition, from a Preternatural Dilation of a Bag Formed in the Pharynx," *Medical Observations and Inquiries* 3: 85. Society of Physicians London, 1769.

Zenker, Friedrich Albert von and Herbert von Ziemssen. "Krankheiten des Oesophagus." In Volume 7, supplement, *Handbuch der Speciellen Pathologie und Therapie.* edited by Herbert von Ziemssen, 1-87. Leipzig, 1877.

Chapter Twelve

Brewer, Lyman. "The First Pneumonectomy: Historical Notes," *Journal of Thoracic and Cardiovascular Surgery* 88 (1984): 810-826.

Churchill, Edward D. and Ronald Belsey. "Segmental Pneumonectomy in Bronchiectasis," *Annals of Surgery* 109 (1939): 481-499.

Macewen, William. "The Cavendish Lecture: Some Points in the Surgery of the Lung," *British Medical Journal* 2 (1906): 3-7.

Ochsner, Alton. "The Development of Pulmonary Surgery, with Special Emphasis on Carcinoma and Bronchiectasis," *American Journal of Surgery* 135 (1978): 732-746.

Zhang, Sarah. "The Surgeon Who Experimented on Slaves." *Atlantic Monthly,* April 2018. https://www.theatlantic.com/health/archive/2018/04/j-marion-sims/558248.

Chapter Thirteen

Brewer, Lyman. "The First Pneumonectomy: Historical Notes," *Journal of Thoracic and Cardiovascular Surgery* 88 (1984): 810-826.

Brewer, Lyman. "Historical Notes on Lung Cancer Before and After Graham's Successful Pneumonectomy in 1933," *American Journal of Surgery* 143 (1982): 650-659.

Churchill, E.D., R.H. Sweet, L. Soutter and J.G. Scannell. "The Surgical Management of Carcinoma of the Lung," *Journal of Thoracic Surgery* 20 (1950): 349-365.

D'Amico, Thomas A. "Historical Perspectives of the American Association for Thoracic Surgery: Evarts A. Graham," *Journal of Thoracic and Cardiovascular Surgery* 142 (2011): 735-739.

Ellenberg, Jordan. *How Not to be Wrong: The Power of Mathematical Thinking.* New York: Penguin, 2014.

Graham, Evarts A. and J.J. Singer. "Successful Removal of an Entire Lung for Carcinoma of the Bronchus," *Journal of the American Medical Association* 101 (1933): 1371-1374.

Horn, Leora and David H. Johnson. "Evarts A. Graham and the First Pneumonectomy for Lung Cancer," *Journal of Clinical Oncology* 19 (2008): 3268-3275.

deKoning, Harry J., C. M. van der Aalst, P. A. de Jong, et. al. "Reduced Lung Cancer Mortality with Volume CT Screening in a Randomized Trial," *New England Journal of Medicine* 382 (2020): 503-513.

Macewen, William. "The Cavendish Lecture: Some Points in the Surgery of the Lung," *British Medical Journal* 2 (1906): 3-7.

Mueller, C. Barber. *Evarts A. Graham: The Life, Lives and Times of the Surgical Spirit of St. Louis.* Hamilton, ON: B.C. Decker. 2002.

Ochsner, Alton. "The Development of Pulmonary Surgery, with Special Emphasis on Carcinoma and Bronchiectasis," *American Journal of Surgery* 135 (1978): 732-746.

Williams, Harley. *Doctors Differ: Five Studies in Contrast.* London: Jonathan Cape, 1946.

Chapter Fourteen

Adams, W. E. and D. B. Phemister. "Carcinoma of the Lower Thoracic Esophagus: Report of a Successful Resection and Esophagogastrostomy," *Journal of Thoracic Surgery* 7 (1938): 621-632.

Barrett, Norman R. "The Lower Esophagus Lined by Columnar Epithelium," *Surgery* 41 (1957): 881-894.

Belsey, RHR. "Palliative Management of Esophageal Carcinoma," *American Journal of Surgery* 139 (1980): 789-794.

Earlam, Richard, J.R. Oesophageal Squamous Cell Carcinoma: A Critical Review of Surgery 216 (1980): 583-590

Ellis, Harold. "Franz Torek (1861-1938): First Successful Resection of an Oesophageal Tumor," *British Journal of Hospital Medicine* 69 (2005): 529.

Lewis, Ivor. "The Surgical Treatment of Carcinoma of the Oesophagus with Special Reference to a New Operation for Growths in the Middle Third," *British Journal of Surgery* 34 (1946): 18-31.

Logan, Andrew. "The Surgical Treatment of Carcinoma of the Esophagus and Cardia," *Journal of Thoracic and Cardiovascular Surgery* 46 (1963): 150-161.

Marshall, S. F. "Carcinoma of the Esophagus: Successful Resection of the Lower End of the Esophagus with Reestablishment of Esophageal Gastric Continuity," *Surgical Clinics of North America* 18 (1938): 643-648.

McKeown, K. C. "Total Three-Stage Oesophagectomy for Carcinoma of the Oesophagus," *British Journal of Surgery* 63 (1976): 259-262.

Pompei, Mario F. and James B.D. Mark. "The History of Surgery for Carcinoma of the Esophagus," *Chest Surgery Clinics of North America* 10 (2000): 145-151.

Skinner, David B., Alex G. Little, Mark K. Ferguson, Alfonso Soriano and Vicki M. Staszek. "Selection of Operation for Esophageal Cancer Based on Staging," *Annals of Surgery* 204 (1986): 391-401.

Torek, Franz. "The First Successful Resection of the Thoracic Portion of the Oesophagus for a Carcinoma," Surgery, Gynecology and Obstetrics 16 (1913): 614-617.

Chapter Fifteen

Cerfolio, Robert J., Jose Ribas Milanez de Campos, Ayesa S. Bryant, Clidd P. Connery, Daniel L. Miller, Malcolm M. DeCamp, Robert J. McKenna and Mark J. Krasna. "The Society of Thoracic Surgeons Expert Consensus for the Surgical Treatment of Hyperhidrosis," *Annals of Thoracic Surgery* 91 (2011): 1642-1648.

Dermatologic Clinics of North America. *Hyperhidrosis.* Edited by David M. Pariser, volume 32, issue 4. 2014.

Chapter Sixteen

Woolf, Virginia. *On Being Ill.* Ashfield, MA: Paris Press, 2002.

About the Author

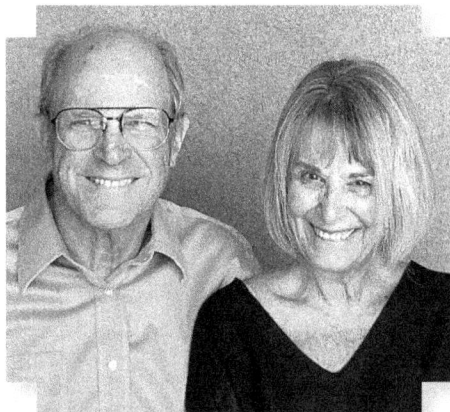

Dr. Alex Little has spent his career as an academic general thoracic surgeon. He graduated from Johns Hopkins Medical School and trained in surgery both at Hopkins and the University of Chicago. Subsequently, he was a faculty member in Chicago before acting as chair of the Departments of Surgery for the Universities of Nevada and Wright State (Ohio). Dr. Little also served as President of the American College of Chest Physicians.

His career overlaps with a time of rapid growth for general thoracic surgery—surgery for the lungs, esophagus, and other chest organs. He has worked with and knew many of the surgeons instrumental in the development of the specialty. As a lifetime teacher of students and residents and practitioner of thoracic surgery, he has the perspective and experience to tell the story of the origins and development of this specialty.

In retirement, he lives in Tucson with his wife, who dazzles him every day.

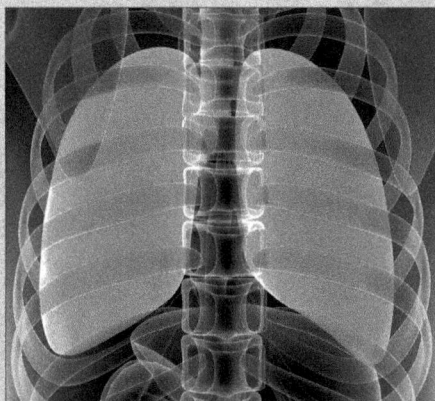

Cracking Chests

How Thoracic Surgery Got from Rocks to Sticks

Alex G. Little, M.D.

Author website: alexlittlemd.com

Available through:

Ingram

Amazon

BN.com

SDPPublishing.com

SDP Publishing

Contact us at: info@SDPPublishing.com

www.ingramcontent.com/pod-product-compliance
Lightning Source LLC
Chambersburg PA
CBHW070839100426
42813CB00003B/683